The Hand I Was Dealt

Essential Tremor

Greg's Story

By

Greg Northover

Steven Northover

Copyright ©2020

AlwaysHeadingNorth.com

Introduction

We wrote this book to help others understand and cope with essential tremor. Essential tremor usually begin slowly. One day at a time, others around us notice we tremble. Sometimes they stare or make comments. We don't understand what is wrong with us. We make excuses. Or we withdraw.

We don't need to be embarrassed. We do need to understand.

As trembling increases, our misbehaving bodies rob us of our ability to do the things we enjoy. We can no longer use hand tools as we once did. Our handwriting, once excellent, begins to resemble scribbling. And worse, some of us lose the ability to do the simplest things like tie our shoes, button our buttons, pour a drink, or eat without spilling somewhere between our plates and our mouths.

We think we are alone. No one else we know is like us.

We are not alone. In the United States, our best estimate is four percent of us have essential tremor. Let's round the number to ten million of us. We are a big group. When we add in the people who care about us and, in some cases, provide care, the numbers of people who are affected doubles.

The first half of this book tells a story about one couple, Greg and Sue. Greg trembles. Sue helps him cope. He trembles so bad he was laid off and needs help with most daily activities. While we highlight him, he could not manage without her. Sue is the unsung hero.

The second half of this book covers other conditions people who have essential tremor frequently discover they have. We offer the knowledge we have gleaned and some approaches some found helpful in dealing with these other problems.

Who Should Read This Book?

Three broad classes of people should read this book. First, are the people who know or suspect they have essential tremor. This book was written specifically for you. You may be young. We know of a few people who are not yet teens who tremble. You will find information here that will help you.

You may be in the middle of your life. Many of us begin to tremble in our late 30s or early 40s. Well-intentioned acquaintances may ask if we are cold or suggest we should cut back on the coffee. Some may imply we are drinking too much alcohol. We may have no idea why we shake. Nor do we know what we can do about it. Eventually, we may decide to ask our doctor. We wrote a portion of this book to help you get ready to have that discussion.

You may be retired. Essential tremors don't go away. In general, as we age, our tremors grow worse. You can find ways to cope, to stay engaged with life, and to accept yourself.

For tremblers of every age, people with essential tremor, we must find ways to cope. As tremors steal our abilities, we must search for new ways to live and new things we enjoy doing.

The second group includes the people who live with someone who has essential tremor. You may be a spouse or a parent. You will want to understand what the one who trembles is experiencing. Some trembling days are worse than other days. The tremblers may have trying days with frustration, disgust, anxiety, sadness, depression, or even despair. We, tremblers, may long for the days when we were "normal." We may have days when we are hard to live with.

Helping someone who trembles can be hard work. Tremblers and our helpers must find ways to prevent exhaustion and burn-out.

Third, we hope some doctors, general practitioners, primary care physicians, and nurses will spend an hour or two reading this book. You may recognize the essential tremor's earliest stages in your patients before they do. You will be in a better position to help your patients understand what is happening to them.

Dedication

We dedicate this story to all the tremblers, the people who have movement disorders.

In a game of cards, "the hand you were dealt cannot be changed, but the way you play it can.

Successify.net/2013/04/24/playing-the-hand-youre-dealt

Thanks to all the people who helped design the cover and who offered early reader comments. We know lists like this are usually written first name first. We wanted it to be very easy for contributors to find their names.

Agans, Ed **Albertson**, Carrie **Albertson**, Laura **Bates**, Cheryl **Bonds**, Venita and Byron **Broward**, Gordon **Brown**, Jeff **Burk**, Diane **Butcher Baker**, Pearl **Carnegie**, Charlotte **Crafton**, Cindy **Bryant DaVita**, Helen **Deseke**, Sandra **Easter**, Lauren **Franco**, Mary Smith **Hadler Baines**, Jessica **Hayter**, Julie **Lane**, Mike **Leh-Pargac**, Debbie **Lentz**, Sarah **Mackelprang**, Cindy **Marquez**, Alba Irene **Mitchell**, Gaby **Northover**, Jennifer **Northover**, Michael **Ockene**, David **Ridgway**, Mary **Seeley**, Tracey **Shelton**, Sue **Skaggs**, Larry **Stewart**, James, and Dianne **Wilson**, Paula **Witty**, Kathy Clawson **Yeagley**, Marianne McClain and **Zemla**, Sharon.

Cover 3D brain image used with permission: This cover has been designed using resources from Freepik.com. kjpargeter created the brain image.

Forward

Life is like a card game. Greg's hand included a movement disorder card called essential tremor (ET). He had better cards. High-value cards, including a pleasant, cheerful, optimistic personality. Plus, he had cards for strength, endurance, and height.

Greg's life's journey is like all who have movement disorders. In the first half of his life, he did not know he was living with the potential to experience essential tremor. It stayed submerged and went unnoticed. Then, gradually, his damage accumulated. His awareness grew. Like most of us, he disregarded his growing symptoms for a time. Essential tremor, having emerged, began to change everything.

His life changed for the worse as he trembled more often. Each of us can learn from Greg's example. Despite a lay-off, his inability to find a new job, and his total disability due to tremors, he never stopped living, enjoying life, and moving forward.

We can learn much from Greg about living with movement disorders like essential tremor and for coping with the other related problems people have.

Table of Contents

About the Authors

Greg has more than fifteen years of experience dealing with debilitating levels of essential tremor. His experiences are the basis for the first half of this book.

Steven loves reading, researching, and writing. His favorite topics include movement disorders, medicine, medical research, cannabis and psychoactive drug research, and history, both military and political. He first became aware of his movement disorder, essential tremor, about 30 years ago.

Also by Steven Northover:

Disasters, Catastrophes, and the End of the World.

information contained within this document, including, but not limited to, errors, omissions, or inaccuracies.

Chapter One: A Layoff!

Thank God, it's Friday!

Greg arrives every day about a half-hour before starting time. "Getting ready for the workday is a great part of my day. I take off my street shoes. Then I slip into my coveralls. If the weather is cold, I protect my feet with heavy wool socks. Otherwise, I put on lighter-weight tube socks. Then I snug my feet into my steel-toed boots. I grab my safety glasses, hard hat, and finish up with leather gloves. Then I head out to the yard," he recounted. "I come in early and leave on time. I never called in sick!"

Greg drives his forklift toward its parking spot in the warehouse. Today, unlike the early days, it was a light workday. Many days people and companies brought in their scrap metals all day long. Less than a dozen people brought in their scrap metals today. It was the same yesterday. "It has been more than a month since we were busy," he thought.

Greg's workday is over. Looking around the copper storage warehouse, he sees a growing problem. Its once full copper scrap bins are nearly empty. His brow furled and lips closed tight, he breathes in deeply. The heavy copper metallic smell he enjoys still lingers, faintly.

The warehouse, completely open inside, amplifies and echoes the forklift's steady engine noise. The yard has about a dozen forklifts and bobcats for handling the scrap metal. The noisy diesel engines pump out a heavy, dull, annoying, lingering, clinging odor. Greg slowly and cautiously maneuvers his noisy forklift into its spot. To his left and right, the other forklifts and bobcats are haphazardly parked. The forklifts are all here. Some of the bobcats are still in the yard. His right hand trembles as he reaches toward the key. His hands tremble now whenever he does things.

For a moment, Greg thinks of his great loves; trucks and mud hopping. There is nothing better than a big, old, noisy truck with big tires and lots of power thrashing the mud and splashing it all over. "Sue doesn't ever get in. She hates the climb. Sue needs a ladder to climb in." Greg chuckles.

Parked, he shuts off the engine. The warehouse becomes quiet. He pulls the key out of the ignition. He looks around once and then steps lightly out of the forklift. As he turns to head to the office where the key is secured overnight, he sees the yard manager and waves and nods his direction. Greg, a tall, friendly man, gets along well with everyone. Even his managers.

The yard manager waves. "Leave the key in the forklift, Greg. Head on over to the main office. They want to see you. I'll take care of this."

Greg nods. He looks himself over, and thinks, "I guess I look okay. I wonder what this is about?"

Things had been peculiar for the past week. Greg noticed the yard and the main manager looking him over attentively. "I wonder what they are doing," he questioned? "Maybe this meeting will clear that up."

Greg confidently strides toward the office. It is quiet. Upon reaching the main office, he opens the door and peers inside. "Payroll. That can't be good," he thinks. All the top scrap yard managers are inside. All five. But not the owner. Greg, who is never one to be nervous, inhales slowly and steps inside. The wood floor squeaks beneath his work boots. Self-consciously he checks to make sure he tracked nothing in.

"Close the door, Greg. Come in. Take a seat." His manager waves toward a chair. Greg sits first. The five managers still standing then take their seats.

"Greg, the last couple of months, we have seen a downturn in the market. People aren't bringing in their scrap metal. The market for scrap is soft. We don't have enough work to pay the bills. We don't have enough work to keep you busy."

"Can you move me to some other job in the yard?" Greg asks.

Greg's manager thinks for a moment, then continues, "We are laying off just about everyone. We filled the few positions we are keeping."

Greg's neck muscles hurt. His teeth clench. His face flushes red. "I'm one of the best workers you've got," he thought, almost out loud. But he keeps his thought to himself. His anger dissolves. His head bows. He lightly touches his forehead with his calloused thumb and fingertips. Greg's eyes close.

"We've got to let you go, Greg," his manager said matter-of-factly. The room grew quiet. The managers, all five of them, were uncomfortable. One manager shifted in his seat. Someone coughed.

"Greg," his manager says softly. "I can't read your weight tickets. You shake all the time. I am sorry. I am."

Greg nods. "I don't know what it is. Just the shakes, I guess. I don't do drugs. I never have. I'm a good worker — one of your best. You know I am. I've been working here for years."

His manager responds, "I know. You can draw unemployment while you look for work."

Greg's shoulders drop. His lungs fill with air. He sits up tall, all six feet one hundred eighty-five pounds of him. Straight. Hard. "Okay," Greg said. Greg's eyes meet his manager's eyes. Kind, friendly eyes briefly hold his gaze. Slightly embarrassed, his manager looks away.

The HR manager, Greg, never could remember her name, passes a small buff manila folder she has been holding to Greg's manager.

"I have papers for you to sign, Greg," he says. Then I can get you paid."

And just like that, it is over.

For a moment before standing up to leave, Greg thinks about it, then decides to speak. "Well, sometimes bad things happen." He spoke clearly, directly and decisively to the assembled managers.

Each manager stood, stepped toward Greg, extended their hands to shake his, then thanked him for his work. "Thanks, Greg. I am sorry this happened. Good luck!"

Greg stood, shook hands, then left to pack his things. "I feel numb. Well, I won't be coming back here," he thought. Surprised at this turn of events, he thought of nothing else as he walked from the Main Office building to the locker building to pick up his things. "Laid off! Now what?"

Greg bunched up his rain gear, including a raincoat, rain pants, and a second pair of boots. He turned toward the exit. Before he left the locker building, two co-workers stopped him. "What's going on, Greg?" He wasn't the only one laid off that day. He wasn't the first. Nor was he the last. Others, worried, noticed.

"It has been really nice working with you," Greg said and smiled. "See you another day." It was a great crew. "They were all really nice," he thought. "I'm gonna miss the practical jokes. I always gave as good as I got."

"What about Sue?" Greg wonders. "What should I tell her? Was I just laid off? Or was I fired? No. The company just laid me off. Now, what will I do? What will we do? What will Sue think?" he asks himself. Greg, a man who can talk to anyone about anything, had no idea how he would tell Sue.

"What a way to start the weekend," he mumbles. Greg, trembling, looks around the yard one last time. "This scrap metal yard was a good place to work." When he first started, the whole job involved separating and sorting the scrap metal. One day the yard manager asked him if he could run one of the forklifts. "What a day that was," Greg thought. After that, he ran forklifts, Bobcats, the front loader, and the excavator. Even later, the yard manager asked him to help load trucks. Greg smiled, sadly, as he thought if it. "There is an art to loading trucks. Each truck is different. But now, they can't read my tickets. I can't either."

"I'm gonna miss this place, the noise, the smells, and the people too, I s'pose," he said quietly to himself. "Especially the people." Saddened, Greg turned back toward his truck.

His drive home begins at the scrap metal company in the Tacoma Tide Flats. It ends fifteen long minutes later at an apartment complex on Pacific Avenue.

"Well, crap." Greg thought back to when he started working at the scrap yard. It was a cold, dreary, gray winter day in 2005. "Seven and a half years ago." Not at all like today.

"Pretty day out." It is a Pacific Northwest sunny day. Nice. Warm.

"I have to get another job," Greg says out loud to no one. "And sign up for unemployment."

Outside his apartment, he fiddles with his door key. Some days the tremors make it tough to put the key in the lock. His right hand bounces around wildly. Greg's hands and arms dance as he positions the key. "C'mon. Settle down. Damn it! Hit the hole." On the third try, the key finds the lock. He turns the key clockwise and opens the door.

Sue is already home. He steps in and closes the door behind him. "They laid me off, Sue."

"Living here takes two incomes, Greg," Sue said softly. She looked at him. She didn't say anything else.

"I'll go to the Lakewood unemployment office first thing on Monday," Greg replies.

"Okay," Sue said. "I'll make dinner."

"I will put my stuff away," Greg says as he heads toward one of the bedrooms. After he puts his work things away, he changes out of his work clothes. Greg looks at his trembling hands. "It's pretty bad today," he thinks.

"I just gotta wash my hands," Greg yells through the door to Sue. "I'll be there in a minute." As he reaches for the soap dispenser, he knocks it over. It goes right off the counter, clattering loudly and breaking on the floor. "Oh crap, another mess to clean up," he says quietly.

While Greg cleaned things up, he thought about Sue. They met long ago. Sure, Greg liked her from the beginning. While Greg was sure Sue liked him, she had a boyfriend and a problem. She needed a place to stay for a couple of weeks. Greg offered the couch in his living room. A month passed. Greg and Sue gradually did more things together. Sue never mentioned her boyfriend, who faded away. Over time others saw them as a couple. And then they saw themselves as a couple. They started doing everything together, including working together. "We argued once. It was over a beer. I wanted one. Sue didn't like that. Other than that, we just don't argue with one another," Greg thought and smiled.

Greg pushes his food all around the plate. Losing his job is a grave setback for both of them. And then there are his worsening tremors. Both toy with their food in silence. Greg finally breaks the silence, "It won't be hard to find work. Someone needs a Bobcat or forklift operator. Or maybe a truck driver. I drove a truck for the Goodwill once. I used to run around Tacoma, picking up the trash bins. Remember?"

Sue's eyebrows raised.

Greg smiles. It is his first real smile since he left the managers in the company's main office an hour ago. He continues, "Drivers called 'em trash bins. People throw their trash in 'em."

"I don't want you to drive long haul again," Sue said. "I don't think your eyes are good enough anymore," she continued. Greg paused, thinking, "Yeah, she'd miss me."

"I wonder who needs a forklift or Bobcat operator?" he asked. "I don't know," Sue replied. Each one, in a prison of their own making, wondered how they would make ends meet. Neither one spoke if it.

Greg noticed Sue watching him tremble.

It was not a happy weekend.[1]

Chapter Two: Paperwork

Monday morning finally came.

Greg and Sue drove to Lakewood. Neither one spoke. At 5'5" tall, Sue is a generous half foot shorter than Greg. She worries enough for both of them, but mainly, she worries about him.

"There it is," he says. "The unemployment office is in that group of buildings. It sorta looks like a small community college campus." He parks his truck. He and Sue walk past the trees toward the entrance. She squeezes his hand briefly, then he opens the door, and both enter. There are plenty of people inside. Greg waits patiently for his turn.

Sue picks up the paperwork and a clipboard. Greg's hands are shaking. He shakes all the time now. Greg's tremors have worsened over the last few years. Greg pretends to be happy, but Sue knows better. Sue fills out the government forms while they wait. It is the first step in the government's process. After a long wait, a clerk calls Greg's number. She quickly looks through his paperwork, while reciting the rules Greg will follow. That is it.

Greg enthusiastically looks for businesses with openings. He worked for Goodwill before. He drove a truck for them. But this time, it didn't work out. These days drivers need a Commercial Driver's License, and Greg doesn't have one anymore. "With my shakes, I couldn't fill out the logbooks anyway," he thinks.

Over the next month, Greg applies for a dozen jobs each time in person. Everyone says, "No."

Greg shakes pretty bad. It doesn't take much to see him shaking. His handwriting is unreadable. His arms and hands are the most noticeable. And every potential employer somehow finds some other applicant who is a better fit for their open position.

Greg keeps looking. Sue, always patient, always supportive, worries.

One evening Sue asks, "Are you cold, Greg?" "Uh, no," he replies. "Why?

"Your head is shivering," Sue responds. "It looks like you are shaking your head no."

"I don't know," Greg said. It was equal parts question and answer. "I wish this never happened. I can't do things I should be doing. I'm pissed. Why can't I find a job? Why won't anybody hire me?"

Greg sighed. Sighs come more often these days. "Anyway," Greg says quietly, trailing off.

The State unemployment office approved Greg's claim quickly. It was not enough to cover the rent. While Greg kept looking for work, Sue filled the gap. She held down three different part-time jobs. He applied for every open position he learned of. But he never found work. Both waited to see what would come next. Sue and Greg would struggle to stay even for the next four years.

"Greg, I think you need to apply for disability," Sue said. "It has been more than a year now. Every place you applied to has told you no." "I want to work, Sue. I'm not disabled. I shake a little," he responds.

"You shake a lot. People see it," Sue replies gently. "How many places did you go to in person? Fifty? Seventy-five? A hundred?"

"Yeah, about that," Greg admits.

"We need the money, Greg. I am doing all I can. Even with three part-time jobs, we don't have enough. We are juggling bills. Unemployment is going to run out sooner or later," Sue, the practical one, nudges him. "C'mon. Let's see what we need to do. I'll go with you."

Greg admits, "I don't know why I can't find a job. It's depressing." He looks at Sue. Her expression is soft. Caring. Even concerned. But her eyes have a hard edge. Greg continues, "Maybe you're right about jobs. You work three jobs. You are a caregiver and works concessions at the Tacoma Dome. And, yeah, you're a good bartender and short-order cook. And I can't find one job. It's been more than a year. It's September."

Greg's lips pressed hard together. "I will look up disability."

Disability

"Sue," Greg said, "While you were working, I looked up disability. We have to go to the Social Security Office over by the Mall."

"Oh yeah. Over by the Tacoma Mall," Sue comments. As she turned to look at Greg, her long, blond hair fell across her face. She tucked it behind her left ear.

"There's going to be paperwork. I can't fill out the paperwork anymore," he tells Sue.

"I'll fill it out for you, Greg. I'll take some time off, and we'll go," Sue replies.

They went the next morning.

Sue and Greg sat in silence on the bus on the way over. There was not much to say. His face flushed. He was embarrassed. "I can't fill in forms by myself. No one can read my writing. Not even me," he thought. "Thanks for coming with me, Sue," Greg said.

"It's okay, Greg."

It took a long walk, twenty minutes or so to get to the bus stop. Then an hour ride on two different busses with a transfer in between. The second bus stopped at the bus terminal near the Mall.

"Let's do this." Sue squeezes his hand. As the bus driver opens the door, Greg turns to Sue and nods, "Okay." Three steps down and both are on the sidewalk. Greg points out their destination, "I think it's this way, Sue."

Greg closes his light jacket. It is chilly out. In another hour or two it will be comfortable. It is about two blocks to the social security office. Greg, in no hurry, walks with even steps. Sue pulls him forward toward their goal. "I guess that's it," he says. "Over there, across the parking lot. The lot's already full. I bet we have to wait."

They both look across the small but full parking lot at the low, one-story brick building. Solid, raised gold letters, "Social Security Administration" on the outside wall facing the lot mark their destination.

Fifty steps later, they were standing at the end of the line. Greg did a quick headcount. "Thirty people ahead of us. People bring their kids. Amazing."

Security was tight. Once inside, they waited their turn to go through the airport-style metal detector. You know the drill. Things go in a bin. Belts come off. Electronic devices checked. Then inside. Next–a touch screen. Sue types in Greg's social security number. "There are two seats over there, Greg," Sue says. She picks up a clipboard, black government pen, and the typical government form.

Then they sat. Sue filled in the information the government form asked. There were a couple of pages, three maybe. Then they waited. And waited. And waited.

Eventually, the display pops up Greg's number and gives him the window number. Sue set down the clipboard, dropped the pen in a wire cup filled with other black pens, then handed the clerk the paperwork. The woman on the other side of the window looked over his form and decided it was okay. "This looks complete. We will send you a letter with an appointment date," she said. "The letter will have a case number and your adjudicator's name." The woman dismissed them.

At least the weather is cooperating. Most September mornings are crisp. By the middle of the day, the temperature is comfortable. Today the sky is clear. No rain. Greg and Sue walk two blocks to the bus terminal. This time they wait for half an hour for their bus at the terminal. Then a half-hour ride, a wait of about an hour, a transfer, and a second bus ride. And then they walk the rest of the way home.

"I should see a doctor," Greg mentioned to Sue. "Good idea. I will take some time off so we can go together," Sue replied. It was time to get some medical attention. A few days later, they walked together to a nearby neighborhood clinic. A Physician's Assistant (PA) spoke with them, asked lots of questions and took lots of notes. Both Sue and Greg answered the PA's questions. The PA talked to the doctor. When the PA returned, she told Greg and Sue the doctor believed Greg had essential tremor. Sue kept her thoughts to herself. The doctor prescribed Propranolol and recommended a follow-up appointment with a neurologist. While Propranolol is used for other things, it is frequently used to treat tremor symptoms. Greg took it only to discover one of its side effects, an urgent need to urinate, was too much for him to handle. The doctor took him off Propranolol.

Then the trial and error phase began. Primidone was next. Again, the side effects were worse than trembling. It can be hard to find the right drugs and doses. Some people never find a good combination. In turn, Greg tried a half dozen other drugs, and each had troubling side effects. So, Greg went without.

Greg's tremors worsened, as tremors often do. Greg's frustrations rose. And Sue noticed every time. "Do you need some help, Greg?" she would ask. "Yes, please!" But sometimes Greg gratefully responded, "I need to try harder first."

Usually, Sue figured things out and simply did many day-to-day things for Greg.

Week after week, Greg looked for work. He looked nearly every day. He applied in person for every job opening he found for a truck driver, forklift operator, or Bobcat operator. With his years of experience and a good recommendation from the scrap metal company, Greg knew his next job was "just a matter of time." But bills must be paid. Sue kept working her three jobs while watching every penny. Even with government assistance, some cash and food stamps, they were not making it.

Greg kept looking for work. Months passed. Eventually, he looked at every open job. In hindsight, his tremors were a problem. People with tremors figure it out. Every employer found someone better suited for their open positions. The times were hard. Greg and Sue had to walk to the food bank. Living was difficult. Yet Sue and Greg somehow kept their positive attitudes.[1]

The social security administration denied Greg's claim three times. It took three years before Greg went before an administrative judge. A Department of Transportation administrator advised the judge who declared Greg completely disabled.

Chapter Three: The Move

As often happens in life, things changed.

"Greg, the owners sold the apartments." "They said they might," he responded.

Sue held out a notice. "They are raising our rent, Greg. A hundred dollars. We don't have another hundred dollars." "I guess we'll have to find another place," Greg said quietly.

Sue pauses. She says, "Oh, Jennifer called. Zodiac is hiring."

"How is your daughter doing? And her husband, Jason?" Greg asks.

"Okay. We talked. Jennifer thinks I should apply. Zodiac's a big company in Newport. If they hire me, we'll have to move," Sue replied.

Zodiac hired Sue. Jennifer offered to let Sue and Greg come live with them for a couple of months while they looked for a place to live. Sue put together a quick yard sale. Greg and Sue sold everything they could. What they couldn't take to Newport, they put in storage. In June 2015, they said farewell to Tacoma and hello to Newport.

Newport, Washington. If you stand on the edge of town and stroll toward the east, you can be in Idaho in five minutes. People say the elevation and the population are the same. The truth is the elevation is 2,160 feet. Newport's population at that time was 2,170 people.

Canada is one hour north by car.

Sue worked for Zodiac Aerospace. About a hundred people worked there. They make things for the aircraft cabins. Sue started working there at the end of June.

Timing is everything. It is the Fourth of July! Independence Day. Picnics. Hot dogs. Soft drinks. Beer. Laughter. And fireworks. Jennifer, Jason, their three children, Sue and Greg, packed up some sandwiches, soft drinks, a little bit of beer, and headed off to the town of Priest River in Idaho.

Every year Priest River hosts a picnic and fireworks at Bonner Park West. The people call it the Docks. It is a small park overlooking the Pend Oreille River. In case you were wondering, the river is pronounced pond oh ray. It seems some French-Canadian fur trappers gave the river its name. That was about 200 years ago. The name stuck.

The park is not too big. It has some barbeque pits under a covered area, restrooms, a couple of picnic tables, a swing set, plenty of grass, and a dock on the river. But it's beautiful. A fence separates the park from the parking lot. Between the grass and the water, there are about 30 feet of river sand.

Before special events like Independence Day, an older, retired couple drive in and stay in their comfortable recreational vehicle. They try to be helpful. They watch over the place.

Jennifer and Sue laid out a big blanket. Greg and Jason carried the cooler with the sandwiches, soda, and beer. The kids ran down to the half-moon dock. It's not really a half-moon. The park is on the north side of the river. On the east side of the park, the dock runs straight into the water for at least 80 feet. The engineers designed a crisp ninety-degree turn toward the west. The dock runs another 80 feet. To make the best use of the space, the engineers angled the dock back toward the shore at about 120 degrees.

The engineers built four slips for small boats on the side facing the river. Then the dock has one more lazy turn back toward the shore. The dock forms a big safe space on the river. The kids can't be dragged away by the river. Most parents think that's a good thing.

For the kids, this will be a day of jumping in the water, swimming, splashing, running back and forth, eating sandwiches and drinking sodas. For the adults, it is about the same. Well, except for the jumping in the water, swimming, splashing and running back and forth. And the adults can have a beer or two if they want.

For the adults, this is an afternoon for small talk, some jokes, storytelling, a little bit of eating, and some drinks. And carefully watching their kids. Everyone helps themselves to the sandwiches and drinks.

Greg carefully picks up his sandwich with both hands. He looks it over. Bread, of course. Cheese. Bologna, lettuce, a tomato, and mayo. Before tremors, he never thought about how his body picks up a sandwich, with just the right amount of force to keep it together without squishing out the contents. Those days are over.

"It helps if I focus on my sandwich. Both hands. Slow. Don't hold it too tight. Now up to my mouth. Don't squish it!" Sometimes it works. Usually, it doesn't.

Sometimes other people stare. Sometimes it's the kids. They quickly notice the young adult making a real mess of his sandwich. The adults see it too. Most, out of pity or politeness, avert their eyes. That is uncomfortable. There isn't much Greg can do about it. He doesn't complain about how life is not always fair. "Thank goodness for Sue. How would I live without her?"

All too soon, the afternoon turns to early evening. The town shoots its fireworks off the docks over the river. Priest River is a little town, and the fireworks display is a small show. Greg lay on his back so he could look mostly straight up. After the usual 30 minutes of "oohs" and "ahs," the show is over. It is time to go back to Washington State and home.[1]

Chapter Four: The Woods, The River, and the Fish

Greg fishes mostly on weekends. He fishes every chance he gets. He loves the water, the woods, and the fish. He often thinks of the many times he fished in The River or out on the ocean. From time to time now, Greg relives those good days. Most of the stories he tells himself are good stories.

"I love the way the water in a creek or river moves. Water flows over rocks. It gurgles and laughs. There is nothing more relaxing than walking through the woods on the way to a creek. In the spring, the plants, trees, nesting birds, and the rest of nature, burst with colors, sounds, and good, soothing smells. All of life's problems melt away as I take step after step through the woods."

Greg's first fishing experiences were in Chambers Creek near where he lived. That was way back in grade school. "Marty, a neighbor boy, ten, the same age as me, brought two fishing poles by one day. You know Marty was deaf, totally deaf," Greg recounted. "But we went anyway. Marty waved the fishing poles around and pointed toward the creek. I nodded, and off we went. Marty waved his hands around when we got to his favorite spot. It was my first time fishing, and it was easier then. A bamboo pole. A bit of line. A hook. And some worms, salmonberries, artificial rubbery worms, it didn't matter. The fish were eager to be caught. Drop the line in, then pull the fish out."

"I loved fishing in Chambers Creek. At first, I only fished a little, now and then," Greg commented. "One day, Marty didn't want to go. So, I went by myself. It's funny, Marty taught me how to fish. I learned to love it. After that, I fished anytime I wanted to. Except for school days."

"I realized I knew where the fish would be season by season. They like the shadows."

"Eventually, I stopped creek fishing. As I grew older, I started looking at rivers. The Nisqually River passed not too far from my house in Roy, Washington. I'd drive a whole five minutes over to Yelm, and park near the dam."

River Fishing

The Nisqually River in Washington State has its origin in the shadow of Mount Rainier. For Greg, Washington's rivers are alive. Rivers move. They dance. They think. They talk. They tease. They have their own smells. Rivers store up knowledge about life. Rivers are wise and patient. Sometimes rivers are gentle. And sometimes they are treacherous and unforgiving.

Every river speaks to the trees in the forest, to the birds, to the wildlife, and even to the plants. The Nisqually River speaks with a cold glacial accent. Its headwaters, not far from Greg's favorite spot, are fed by the glacier on Mount Rainer's southern exposure. The Mountain, tall, rugged, and majestic catches the Pacific Ocean's moisture, which he stores as snow and ice. The Mountain gives The River clean, cold, icy, water gifts every day.

The River's voice matches her waters. Where The River runs over rocks and boulders, her voice is loud, drowning out all other sounds. In other places, The River slows her pace. Her voice is quiet enough; one can hear the trees brushing each other in the breeze. Mostly The River speaks quietly, with subtlety.

Greg, a young man, athletic and physically strong, steps carefully and quietly through the woods. The early morning sun barely breaks through the dense forest. It is still dark in this wood. The ground is wet from the dew. Water squishes out from under his tennis shoes as he carefully works his way down the gentle slope toward the river. Greg is a comfortable six feet tall. He has a two-piece fishing pole in his left hand. He uses his right hand to grab the low tree limbs to help keep him on his feet where the ground dips. Greg learned early on that tennis shoes with rubber soles were better than boots for fishing.

Insects begin to wake up. The forest slowly grows brighter as the sun's elevation increases. Life in the woods becomes noisy. Greg hears the familiar sounds. Clicking. Buzzing. Zipping. Snapping. All around him, he knows there is life unseen by him. The music of the cold, Nisqually River, rushing over the rocks, tells him he is close. The aroma of cold water, mossy rocks, and clean sand compete now with the dark, earthy, pungent, forest bottom smells.

Greg doesn't look much like a fisherman. No hip waders. Definitely no hip waders. Greg commented, "Fishermen slip in the water and drown in those things. Tennis shoes and sturdy Levis are best for fishing." No tackle box. No beer. Instead, he wears an odd belly pack stuffed full of hooks, bobbers, and a couple of fishing flies. Greg made the fishing flies from small bird feathers tied tightly around a hook with lightweight, strong, fine thread.

Deep in his belly pack, there is one jar filled with bright red and orange salmon eggs. Bait. When he uses salmon eggs, he uses a small number 10 hook. The egg completely hides the hook. The tiny, concealed hook surprises the fish and delights Greg.

The fish, for their part in our story, practice nibbling the bait right off the hook. The best of them look forward to the meal the fishermen provide. The fish swim on well-fed and happy. The fishermen are none the wiser.

Every fisherman wears a hat for luck. Don't they? Greg's hat is a droopy, wrinkled Seattle Seahawks cap. As a football fan, he bought a cap with the Seahawks logo on it. He wears it pulled down close to keep the sun out of his eyes. Except in the rain. When it rains, he turns the cap around, so the rain runs somewhere other than down his neck. The hat, now Greg's fishing cap, is already old. The color, once a deep blue has faded. The Seahawks logo is still distinct, although the bill droops a bit. Its edges are just beginning to fray.

Greg knows this narrow trail. He and others have walked carefully down it just often enough to kill the plants that might otherwise reclaim the brown, exposed soil. The path itself beginning up near the road, twists, and turns as it takes him down to the river. Here near the river, the woods crowd the bank. Just ten more steps over moss-covered rocks. Now, only eight more steps and the waters spread out. Just five more steps and sand replaces rock.

Greg made a big splash his last trip out. He slipped right down the bank, skinning away all the moss. He entered the icy water, leading with his feet, his butt sliding right down the bank, coming to rest in the river bottom. But not this day. No matter. Wet or dry, he is here to fish.

"Last time I screwed up. I stepped around a boulder. Careful! Down I went. The moss is clean enough, but right under all that moss, it's muddy," Greg remembers. Now River Mud is not smart. But all mud is clever. It likes nothing more than to work its way from the seat of a pair of jeans all the way up a fisherman's back. Mud is especially apt when the fisherman is wearing a light jacket. When mud moves, it moves quickly! It took only a second or two for the River Mud to get all over his hands, his jeans, his shirt under his jacket, and both jacket sleeves. River Mud even found its way onto his neck and the back of his head.

Greg's Seahawks cap popped right off his head and landed without complaint in The River. The River, always up for a game, took that cap flying downstream faster than Greg could chase it. But The River lost interest quickly. She let his fishing cap, with mud still on it, come to rest at her edge about fifty feet downstream.

Greg looked downstream. His cap hugged the stream bed on his side of the river. Good. He walked carefully down the river until he reached his Seahawks cap. He picked it up. The River, having had her fun, washed the mud clean. She mischievously replaced the River Mud with river sand. The River Mud went happily on its way.

"Oh, boy."

Greg swished his cap in the river until the last of the sand disappeared back into the river. He wrung it out with both hands, then put it back on his head, still wet.

But all that happened the last time.[1]

The Ways of The River

An experienced fisherman, Greg knows the ways of The River. He knows what he seeks this day. The River is home to trout and salmon. The fisherman intends to catch a few of them for this day's meals. Upstream a small dam, maybe twelve feet tall, holds back some of the water. The trail from the road pops out of the woods about 200 yards below the dam. It's a good thing. Greg knows he must stay at least a hundred yards downstream from the dam to fish as the law allows.

He looks the dam over. On both sides, it has broad, flat, shallow concrete stairs covered with running water. "Fish ladders." When the fish head upstream, they run toward the ladders, leaping into the air at the last moment. Salmon and trout use them to get around the dams. Even a young salmon can jump five feet at a time. Greg's seen it himself.

The River, alive, observing, moving, and scheming, uses the tools she has at her disposal to cut her course through sand and rock. The Nisqually River, born at the edge of a glacier, uses gravity and water to move steadily toward her place of destiny far downstream. After a time, The River will reach Puget Sound, where she will join with it, mingle, and merge—a marriage of sorts.

Above The River, in the trees that crowd the banks, birds complain loudly. The crows are the worst complainers. The crows complain about everything. They chatter back and forth to one another—each black, noisy bird warning others and complaining about the fisherman. The fisherman is spoiling their day. Finches and other tiny birds complain as well. But their voices are not too loud, so their complaints are drowned out by the crows.

But a few birds don't complain. The woodpeckers, always busy, always industrious, have little time to complain. They put their heads into their work while disregarding the noisy, bothersome chattering crowd. There are juicy, delicious insects in the tree's wood. It is their job to find and eat them.

The eagle and the osprey lazily circling high above watch the scene unfolding below. They, too, do so without complaint. They know The River and the fish. Like the fisherman, the birds wait patiently for some tasty trout or salmon to make a fatal mistake. The eagle and the osprey have grown wise over countless generations. For all the time they remember, the eagle and the osprey shared The River with the black bears. And now they share The River, and the fish, with men and sometimes with women.

The fish, too, have grown wise. The fish, most of them anyway, take special care to hide in the shadows. Some say the fish like to stay in the shadows cast by bushes near The River's banks. The smartest among them will seek out some broken, fallen tree resting on The River's bottom. The River plays a game with the trees along her shore. She gradually washes away the soil around each tree's roots. At first, the trees remain standing. Sure, some of the tree's roots find themselves in The River's moving waters. The fish learn to swim under the trees, between the tree's roots. There the fish are safe.

As The River washes away more soil, the tree becomes imbalanced. Then the tree falls right into The River. This amuses The River. And delights the fish.

The River is the source of other entertainment. Humans, mostly young, ride small rafts and innertubes for long distances down The River. Sometimes ten to fifteen of them go floating by, making noise, drinking beer, making messes, and scaring the fish away. Greg patiently waits until the young men and women, river partiers, drift, much like fallen leaves on down the river. Then Greg, knowing the ways of the fish, moves upstream following the fish to their next place.

All fishermen know the fishes' secrets. And so too, do the birds.

The River doesn't care about the birds, the fish, the black bears, nor about the fisherman. The fish, the birds, the black bears, and even the fisherman need The River. The River believes it needs nothing.

The River, patient, and always in motion, finds the easiest way to move toward her destiny. Occasionally, The River runs in a straight line. But usually, The River changes directions. She meanders. She accommodates the rocks, the sand, and the trees that sometimes fall into The River. The River is flexible. She bends.

Sometimes The River's bend is big. Then the water moves quickly on one side, the inside of the curve, but slowly on the outside. Fish prefer the slow side when there are shadows.

The fisherman adjusts his fishing hat.

With his cap adjusted, pole in hand, and belly-pack firmly in place, Greg judges The River's depth and speed. He looks carefully along The River's nearside first. He will cast from this side. The nearside is moving quickly, but it is not yet too deep. Then Greg shifts his attention to the far side. He begins his appraisal just a little downstream. He looks for tree roots, for shadows cast by bushes, and for rocks. A fallen tree is best. The fish know they are safe. The fisherman knows they are not.[2]

Greg looks for salmonberry bushes. Its serrated-edged leaves look sharp and sticky. The berries look like a small clump of salmon fish eggs with tiny whiskers. The salmon and trout love them. When the berries ripen enough to drop into The River, they float downstream. The fish chase them. And the fish gobble them up.

"There." The water swirls around in a pool just downstream from a large rock. His eyes sweep the water's surface, moving slowly upstream. The River is a little slower there. Good!

Greg steps into the moving water. "I love the way the cold-water swirls over my feet and around my legs. I love how cold the water feels on a hot day. My tennis shoes let me feel the river bottom. I look for any place where the sun is in my face. Fish fear shadows. I like to slowly sneak up on the fish. I don't think they can smell me. The water makes noises that cover my movements."

Sometimes the water is low and shallow. Other times it is high, deep, and cold. In the story of Goldilocks and the Three Bears, a young girl learned in life, things may be too hot, too cold, too hard, or too soft. For The River, the same applies. It may be too high or too low; too fast and too choppy. Today the water, in perfect Goldilocks fashion, is just right. The young man, having found his spot, moves to where he can cast upstream across the river to the outside of the bend.

For Greg, it is a good day for fishing.[3]

Chapter Five: Before Tremors, Fishing and the Bear

Not every day is a good day. On one morning, much like this morning, our fisherman, fishing before tremors, had an unexpected adventure. Having approached The River, he searched for the right place. As is his habit, Greg moves slowly, quietly, and deliberately downstream.

The River, amusing herself, throws a fine mist upon her banks. Boulders, cold, passive, patient, and maybe just a bit resentful of the Movers in the woods, use the fine mist to set their slippery traps. The Boulders love the mornings the most. A smooth, wet Boulder is the perfect ankle twister in the morning before the sun begins to dry it.

The cautious Movers sniff the cold morning air. Each Mover comes to the River for its own reasons. Some come to drink. Some come to find mates. Some come to eat the berries that grow along The River's banks. And some come to fish. The Movers know about the slippery traps the Boulders set near The River. And so does our fisherman.

With each step forward, Greg avoids the traps. Between his steps, our young fisherman searches The River for shadows, fallen trees, and slow-moving waters. He looks for the next place to step, focused on avoiding the traps. "It has been a while since I was here last," Greg thinks. "This is the fishing season's opening day. It is the first day of river fishing." He checks his watch. "It is about six-thirty." The sun has been up for an hour. The weather is perfect.

The fisherman scans the tree line. And then the river. "A bear!" Greg freezes. A vein in Greg's neck pulses heavily. "Crap." The bear, a black bear, facing slightly downstream, stands in the flowing river. The powerfully built animal is fishing right at the edge of the river.

"Where is the wind? It is in my face. Has the bear smelled me? Don't think so."

"Breathe Greg," he reminded himself.

The River laughed. Two fishers, both Movers, showed up on her banks searching for food. One, a black bear arrived first. He, or she, The River cannot tell, is powerful, observant, and skillful. The bear is hungry and unpredictable. No. The River knows the bear is predictable.

The bear, he, or she, The River doesn't care, stands in the cold, Nisqually River. The bear knows The River. And the bear knows the fish. With one rapid motion, she swoops the fish right out of the water. Upon the bank, the fish go. First one, then another. And another. High above, the eagle and the osprey, watch, envious of the bear below, fishing in The River.

The second Mover, our fisherman, arrived second. Mindful of the traps set by the Boulders, Greg, our fisherman, practically stumbled upon the bear. The Boulders, always patient, showed no disappointment. The birds, always complaining about the fisherman, complained still. The River played fair. The River did not tell the bear about our fisherman. And he, our fisherman, moved slowly, quietly, and steadily away from the bear. As the saying goes, discretion, being the better part of valor, the fisherman while keeping the bear in view, headed back to his truck.

For the bear, it was a good day to fish.[1]

Return to The River

Greg quickly moved back up the trail to his truck. Opening it, he got in, closed and locked the door. "That was scary," he said aloud.

While Greg thought about what to do, he smoked. At that time, he was a smoker. On fishing days, he tried to remember not to light up. He frequently smoked before tremors. And before COPD.

He packed a sandwich for breakfast. Most fishing days, like this one, begin before 6 AM. When he parked here, Greg, forgetting all about his sandwich, headed right on down to the river. That was an hour ago. "I'll have a late breakfast," Greg thought, eyeing his abandoned sandwich.

He thought about the bear. The bear scared him. He thought about the forest. He thought about the birds. He thought about the sunshine. He thought about The River. Greg loved being near The River. She smells wonderful. Or maybe it was the forest smells. And he thought about fishing.

Then he smoked some more.

After a time, some say an hour; some say longer, Greg decided to return to the river. The bear lived in that woods for a long time. The fisherman had never seen the bear before. No doubt, the bear was busy with life and had little time to linger. One hour, more or less, should be enough fishing time for the bear. Armed with that understanding, he opened the truck door, got out, looked around, sniffed the air, and got ready. He reattached his belly pack, grabbed his hat off the front seat, dragged it over his head from back to front, then picked up his fishing rod. A minute later, Greg reached the edge of the forest.

Our fisherman, at that time a smoker, sniffed the fresh forest air. Could he smell the bear? Mostly his nose filled with lingering smoke from his last cigarette. He wasn't smoking now. He paused, looked around, took a few deep, slow, calming breaths, and pushed further into the forest.

Greg feels the slightly springy and slippery narrow dirt path through the flexible rubber soles of his tennis shoes. The smells from the wet, hard-packed dirt wrinkle Greg's nose. Damp soil, even hard-packed, has an odor to it. On some mornings, the odor is pleasant. But not this morning. The stench of dead, rotting plants wafts up from the ground.

Long ago, this forest was thick stands of cedar. Many years ago, loggers cleared away most of the cedar trees. Logging was a big business near The River. Today most of the cedar is gone. And most of the loggers are gone too. But there are still cedar trees in this forest. Plus, pine. Lots of pine. And ferns.

Some people say the woods are like an iceberg. Most of an iceberg is out of sight, below the water's surface. We see the trees growing before us. But there is much we don't see. At least one-half of the woods live below ground. And just like with the iceberg, what lies below us is teeming with life.

Below Greg's feet, unseen and completely unknown, a whole other form of life exists. Fungi. Fun Ji? Fun guy! We choose to say, fun guy. Why? It is pronounced fun gus, not fun jus. The people who know use both pronunciations.

Today we know more about fungi. We have identified about a hundred thousand unique species of this life form that is neither plant nor animal. Our experts, the people who know the most about fungi, say their best guess is fungi have six to seven million species. Most of them benefit us in some ways. Today, for our purposes, the fungi form a "wood wide web" the trees use to communicate with one another. Sometimes the trees send out warnings. And sometimes the trees shop for goods. Sugars. Minerals. The stuff they need and things they are willing to exchange. How that happens is a story for another day.

Greg pauses again. Silent. Still. He peers first down the trail. Then as best he can, he looks between the trees. Indescribable plants fill the spaces between the trees. He knows he can't see much. He listens intently.

If you grew up near a wood, you know the undergrowth fills in the spaces between the trees. Frequently the trees grow close together. Sometimes they stand in small groups of three or four or five all within arm's length of each other. Sometimes a single deep shaft of sunlight breaks through the treetops. Where it touches the ground, small plants with little purple flowers grow. Some people call the little purple flowers fairy slippers. It is Spring, and things are popping.

In other places, Spring brings Bearberries with their olive drab flat, oval leaves, pink flowers, and bright red berries. Greg steps carefully around the pale white flowers. They are short, maybe a half foot tall, and look a bit like a daisy. The flowers are mostly pale white with just a hint of pink.

Mushrooms! There must be fifty different kinds in these woods. Some, like the unpleasant oyster mushroom, grow in clumps on the tree's sides. Greg spots a dull yellow and orange stack of at least a dozen mushrooms on a tree twenty feet off the path. Chicken of the Woods. Sulfur mushrooms. "I'm gonna have to learn more about mushrooms someday," he muses.

Greg continues to walk down the damp path toward The River. He pauses once again for a pleasant smell. Wild onions grow here. He doesn't see them, but he knows they are close. Wild onions smell like the small onions sold in bundles at the grocery store.

At The River, our fisherman looks again for salmonberries. The berries are yellow and orange. Well, they are more orange than yellow. And salmon like the delicious berries. And so, too, does Greg. Salmonberry shrubs crowd along The River, decorating her banks.

"There's one! Well, a dozen at least." The fisherman carefully reaches in to test the berry's firmness. A few might be ripe. "Ah, there's one." Greg plucks just one berry from the bush, blows a small bug off, and plops it in his mouth. It is a little sweet and mildly fragrant. It tastes like a strawberry. No. Maybe more like a blackberry. He can't decide.

Greg loves these woods and The River. It is quiet yet noisy. Every time he comes, he sees different plants. The Salmonberry grows along The River. He likes the Candy sticks, the Licorice Fern, and the wild ginger with its heart-shaped leaves.

Salmonberries have too mild a taste to make great wine. But paired with some other, slightly stronger fruit, it has a chance to be delicious. Maybe strawberry with salmonberries would be good. Some home brewers should give it a try. A couple of shakes of crushed black peppercorns might give it a bit of heat. Hmmm. Yum!

The woods are not Paradise. Oh no. Dangerous animals live here. Dangerous plants, too. Greg knows to avoid the poison oak bushes and the poison ivy that grows up the trees. The poison oak grows in the woods just off the path that begins up by the road where he regularly parks his truck.

Greg stops to listen to The River. The River, murmuring quietly, keeps her secrets. "What will I do if the bear is down by the river again? Run? Any bear can outrun me." Hope would be his strategy today.

The fisherman didn't think the bear would still be there, at his fishing spot. Greg's mind turns to warmth. Once he has his place, he will gather some twigs and dried forest debris and start a small fire near the water's edge.

There is The River now. No bear.

The Brown Trout

On this day, the River played with Greg. She made fun, loud splashing noises as she leaped over the Boulders. Then she stilled her voice as she murmured at the broadest part of a bend. "Come here. The fish wait here," The River whispered in Greg's ears.

He moved over the boulders and a broken tree, its trunk half in the water, half on the bank. His expertise guided by experience led him to keep one hand on the broken tree while he walked in the river. He looked carefully, first down the river, then upstream.

Greg followed the River's voice. He moved to where she beckoned him. Without even looking, knowing it would be there, he adjusted his belly pack. He peered inside to find the right hook, a small number 10 and tied it to his line. Reaching in again, a second time, he found the little jar of salmon eggs. He unscrewed the cap, pulled out one plump egg, and pressed his hook through it. This was a couple of years BT, before tremors.

Greg knows lots about fishing. Naturally, he did everything just right. No one can say for sure how long he had been there, at the river, casting, but suddenly his muscles begin to work. A fish, it was too soon to tell what kind, had hit that egg and jumped right out of the water.

The River, amused, whispered to Greg, "You've got yourself a fat, brown trout if you have the skill to keep her." She laughed. Greg heard The River telling the fish to jump, change directions, and slack the line. This was not the brown trout's first rodeo. She swam hard upstream, jumped in the air then drove hard downstream. If she could make the fisherman's line go slack, it might snag and give her a chance to go free once again. Her strategy worked before. The confident Brown Trout would beat the fisherman. Had it been some other fisherman, she might have won.

It wasn't some other fisherman. Greg knew what to do, and he wanted that fish! The observant River encouraged first

Greg, then the Brown Trout. The River loved playing both sides. She loved the chase. The Contest. The Life and Death Struggle.

He worked his fishing line. "I have to keep it tight."

But not too tight. The Brown Trout swam near the middle of the river. Our fisherman had to drain the energy right out of that fish. The Brown Trout knew she had to make enough slack in the line so she could spit out the hook. Greg knew he had to keep the fishing line tight, well, just right, to keep her hooked. With each change of direction, the fisherman tightened the line a bit more. The Brown Trout swam harder, jumped higher, and changed course. And each time, Greg brought her closer to his side of the river, closer to the bank. And closer to his net.

Ten minutes into the struggle, The River nudged the fish. "Make your move. You are running out of space. You are running out of time."

The Brown Trout, a determined, fierce competitor, changed directions, swimming upstream as fast as she could. She turned, leaped just out of the water then swam quickly toward the fisherman. And the line started to go slack. Just a bit more. The Brown Trout dove toward the bottom. She was going for the snag. She was going for the win.

Greg sensed her strategy in the way the line played with the pole. When she turned and jumped, he was ready. He worked the line, keeping it just tight enough. He held the line taut, even in the turn, in the dive, and the race to the bottom. It was twelve minutes into their contest. The Brown Trout sensed defeat. Greg sensed he had won.

But not yet. The Brown Trout remembered other contests with other fishers. She remembered that other fishermen, who also sensed the turning point grew confident and made little mistakes. And in the end, she had won. In the end, their line sagged. It snagged on debris. She broke free and swam away with full bragging rights.

The Brown Trout repeated her winning strategy four more times. Each time Greg anticipated her timing. Twenty minutes had gone by. The River yawned and looked away. The River knew the fish had lost the contest and her life. The River turned her attention to the Woods, the Movers in the Woods, and the Wind.

Greg noticed the change. The Brown Trout tired. Greg scooped the fish out of the river. He had won. The fisherman carefully took the hook out of her mouth. Eventually, he measured her. Fourteen and a half inches long.

Greg caught two more fish. Catching the brown trout was the best part.[2]

Our fisherman began to think about the sober life and death part of fishing. It was time. Greg thanked the three fish for their sacrifice. Those who hunt and fish to feed themselves will know of this custom. Having praised the fish, he rapidly killed and cleaned them. He selected just one freshly caught trout. He skewered it on a cut, green stick. Then Greg roasted it over his small fire

Chapter Six: The End of Fishing

One day our fisherman had trouble. His fingers trembled more than before. They didn't work quite right for him anymore. He fumbled. Greg focused on the line and the hook. He could not tie the hook to the fishing line. Oh, he had trouble now and then before. In fact, over the last couple of years, his fingers trembled more often. Sometimes he could not tie fishing flies. Sometimes he had trouble tying the hook to the line. Sometimes he could not bait his hook. But this time it was different.

Greg, for the first time, wondered if he might have a problem. He listened to the River. He heard Her voice as The River talked to the boulders, the trees, the birds, and the wind. Everything seemed normal except for his fingers.

Greg paused, then took a deep breath. "Hmmm. Fresh pine! And a hint of cedar," he thought. "Loggers cut most of the cedar down years ago. Maybe there are new trees. Of course, there are new trees," Greg continued his thoughts.

Greg returned to his hook and line. He watched his fingers tremble. Each time he tried to fasten the hook to the fishing line, he failed. Once. Twice. Three times. On his fourth frustrating attempt, he secured the hook to the line. Good! Determination counts.

Greg was nearly ready. He unzipped his belly pack and dug around inside. His fingers knew what to "look" for. After years of weekend fishing, his fingers were second eyes. He wanted the small bottle of fish eggs located deep down at the bottom of his belly pack. There! He unscrewed the cap, reached in, and pulled out a large fish egg. Fish eggs are great bait, but they are a bit tricky to hook.

Ouch! Greg's trembling finger and thumb bounced off the sharp hook's tip. Darn! He dropped the squished egg into the River and sucked the pain out of his pricked thumb. Ugh! The River offered Greg her waters. He bent down near The River, accepting her gift of clear, cold running water. He put his whole hand in up to his wrist. But just for a few seconds. Greg wondered, "What is wrong with me today?"

Then Greg tried to bait his hook again. And again. And again. But Greg's fingers shook, and he could not get the egg on the hook. The eggs squished. Greg looked at his hands. His fingers trembled the way the leaves tremble when the wind gently caresses them. He held his hands out in front of him. His fingers all bounced slightly up and down. Greg's bouncing fingers amused The River but worried Greg. The fish were grateful.

Greg put the last couple of salmon eggs back in his belly pack. He hadn't brought any other bait. Greg wished he'd brought PowerBait. That way, maybe he could make a small ball of that smelly silly putty to put on his hook. Although the last time he brought it, he squished it too. The fish love the darned stuff. To the fish, it smells great and tastes great. But Greg didn't have any. He put his things away. Then Greg looked around himself to make sure he had everything. He took one more look at The River, sniffed the air, took a deep breath, sighed, then slowly shuffled back up the dirt path to his truck. The river, the woods, and most of all the joys of fishing dimmed and darkened.

Last weekend, Greg was a fisher. Today, he is a trembler. Greg's river fishing days have ended.

Greg has essential tremor. His life has changed.[1]

Chapter Seven: Coping With Everyday Life

It's morning.

Bathroom first!

The cats want to be let out first thing in the morning. Then they will play a game of in and out all the rest of the day. "Okay, you little rascals, out you go." Greg softly walks toward the front door. He adjusts his robe and presses his feet deeply into the slippers that give his feet some protection against the cold floor.

Greg doesn't think about tremors. He doesn't have to. His tremors begin when his day begins, although each day is a bit different. On some mornings, Greg's tremors are mild. His fingers hum gently, lightly, so lightly a person without tremors might not notice them.

Most mornings, like this morning, Greg's hands visibly tremble. His fingers bounce up and down together. There is a rhythm to the movements. But each finger also jumps separately. Some fingers move just a little, but others move quite a bit. Greg's cats walk around his feet as he heads toward the door. His cats, smart little animals, manage to avoid being stepped on.

Opening the door is challenging. Greg's left-hand cups the round handle. His thumb and index finger form a sort of funnel. Then his right thumb and index finger reach through the small "O" created by his left hand. Usually, Greg's right thumb makes the first contact with the small "ear" protruding from the center of the lock. A moment, or two, later, his right index finger touches the other side. Success. He turns the small "ear" clockwise that unlocks the door.

The cats are impatient. Greg's door also has a deadbolt. It, too, has an "ear" that must be grasped and turned. More success! The door opens and both cats go tumbling out into the yard. He watches while both cats perform their morning ritual. Emma and Buddy check their territory for intruders as well as for prey. During the night, other animals have come and gone. Some rub against the edges of things to leave their scent. The woods are not that far away. Perhaps a raccoon or two made its way by Greg's door.

"Close the door behind you when you come back in," Greg reminds the cats. Of course, the cats disregard him. It is what cats do. He patiently reasons with his cats every morning. And every morning, his cats push the door open when they are ready to come in. Not once have the cats pushed the door closed behind them.

Greg laughs at the thought of it as he heads into the kitchen.

Cat Breakfast

When the cats come back in, they will want their breakfast. Of course. Greg has a couple of small bags of cat food in his pantry. Picking up the bag is not that much of a problem. Greg grips his right wrist with his left hand. His right hand, steadied somewhat, works well enough to pick up the cat food bag. He sets the bag on the countertop. He retrieves a clean cat bowl from the cupboard. And now the fun begins.

Using both hands, Greg shakes cat food from the bag into the cat bowl. About half ends up in the dish. The rest, thrown about by his trembling hands, falls on the counter. Some kernels land on the floor.

"Sigh," Greg says.

It is the same every morning. Greg tried reaching into the bag, grabbing a fist-full of dry, crunchy cat food. It worked better than pouring. But the cats wouldn't eat the food. So, he shakes the food out of the bag instead.

A cat who won't eat food handled by a person is not especially hungry.

Later in the day, he will feed his cats wet food from a small can. The pull tab is difficult to grasp. Greg mastered a technique. He regularly uses his left hand to steady and guide his right hand. That works well enough for opening cans.

Nothing works well for using spoons. A spoon can be used to scoop food out of a container. But not by Greg. So, he tips the can on its side over the bowl and uses the spoon as a lever to pop the food out of its can and right into the bowl.

Greg's hands and arms begin to tremble harder, faster, and stronger. It is still early. Sue is busy readying herself for work. Most days, she cuts it close. Sue never leaves early. Most days, Sue departs just in time.

"Can you pour me some juice, Sue?"

"Running late, Greg. Outa time!"

" 'kay…"

This morning Sue won't have time to pour him milk, or juice, or water.

Juice

"Well, I can do this," Greg quietly says. Sue bought him a collection of sizeable unbreakable drinking cups with lids. The lids lock tight. Each cover has a straw-sized hole in the middle. Water is the easiest. He begins with water. Greg has a blue cup for water. All Greg's cups are on a shelf in the cupboard. He opens the cupboard door and looks in. The blue cup is in the back.

"I might as well get them all out," Greg says to himself. He grips his right wrist over the top with his left hand. Both hands tremble. "The red cup will do for tomato juice," Greg says to no one in particular. He grips the cup, taking it off the shelf. "That was easy enough." He sets the cup down on the countertop. Greg slides his right hand to the bottom of the cup. The knife-edge of his right hand rests firmly on the counter. Then Greg releases the cup.

Next, Greg repeats the same process with the white cup. He places the cup to the right of the red cup. This time when he let's go, his fingers tap the cup, moving it to the left.

One more time with the blue cup.

With the blue cup in his right hand, he positions his left hand over the cup's lid. His left hand bounces up and down on the cover. Greg's right hand trembles wildly, pushing the cup all over the place. With some difficulty, he lowers the cup to the countertop. Steady now, Greg's left hand grips the lid. A half-twist unlocks the cap.

Greg puts the cup in the sink.

Sue races by the kitchen on her way out. "Bye, Greg. Gotta go!" Sue opens the door. Emma and Buddy race past her, happy to be back in the house. Both cats take an active interest in the drama playing out in the kitchen. Sue closes the door behind her. She will be gone for the day.

"You here to help?" Greg asks Emma. Emma pauses, judges the distance, then effortlessly jumps up on the counter. "Don't knock anything over, Emma. That's my job! Here! Help me with the water."

Greg turns on the cold water. Emma watches the water intensely. "Tell me when the cup is full, Emma." When the cup is 2/3rds full, he turns off the cold water. "Emma! You were s'posed to tell me."

With the cup still in the sink, he puts the lid on. "Would you grab me a straw out of the drawer, Buddy? No? Okay. I will get it myself." Greg carefully picks up one of the big, plastic straws. On the first try, the straw easily slips into the hole in the lid.

"One down. Two to go, Buddy," Greg tells Buddy, his flesh-toned, nearly orange, or maybe more of a buff-colored male cat.

"Shall we do the milk next, Emma? Yes. We shall! Be good, and maybe I will give you some, Emma," Greg says, teasing Emma.

To a casual observer, it might seem surprisingly odd. Greg lifts the water-filled cup out of the sink, replacing it with the white cup. He has a method.

"Do we have any half-gallon cartons of milk left, Buddy?"

Greg opens the fridge door. Buddy helps him look. "No? Too bad. Those are easiest for me to pour. Want to help me with that gallon jug, Buddy?"

Buddy, having already lost interest, sits back down. Greg sets the milk on the counter. The gallon container is still about two-thirds full. It barely bounces around. The weight makes a difference. Milk jugs have plastic screw-on caps. They are small caps. But not too small. One hand steadies and guides the other. After one unsuccessful attempt, Greg grips the cap on the second pass. Good.

Emma helps.

Greg places the milk container on the sink's edge. He uses both hands to line up the milk jug with the cup. Greg pours the milk. Most of the milk goes right into the cup. Most. But not all. About a fifth of the milk splashes into the sink. The cup, about 2/3rds full, is ready. Again, using both hands, he retrieves the cap and, with some effort, gets it back onto the milk jug. Then, repeating the process he used with the lid for his water, Greg locks the top in place, positions another plastic straw in the hole, and lifts the cup filled with cold, delicious milk out of the sink.

One more to go. Tomato juice. Red cup. Sink. Tremors! Splash!

The early morning sun streams in through the kitchen window. Greg's eyes follow the shaft of bright light down to the linoleum floor. The light strikes the kitchen floor about where his tomato juice landed. The liquid sloshed right out of the cup. It sloshed right out of the sink too. Greg's chin dropped. His shoulders slumped. A small sigh huffs out of his mouth. "Crap!" Greg exclaims.

Emma sympathizes a little.

Still, two out of three's not bad.

Greg twists around and reaches for the roll of store-brand paper towels sitting on the counter. "Two sheets ought to do it," he mumbles. Folding them over, he places the sheets under the faucet and turns the water on for just a moment. Then, bending down, he wipes up the splashed tomato juice on the floor. Greg pushes himself up, grabs the counter, and rises to his feet. He turns on the water in the sink and squeezes the juice out. Emma supervises his work. Satisfied with Greg's sink work, she drops to the floor on light cat's paws. Emma sniffs a spot on the floor.

Greg bends back down to check his work. "I see it, Emma."

He captures the last bit of juice in the paper towel. After one last look around the kitchen, and satisfied he found every drop and splash, Greg tosses the still wet paper towel in the garbage can.

"Now, we are ready for the day, Emma."

Greg heads back to the bedroom. Both Emma and Buddy follow. Both want to play. Greg crumples up a ball of paper and tosses it. Both cats run after it and pounce!

"What to wear?" Greg picks up the jeans off the back of the chair. He holds them up, looking them over. "These will do another day."

Greg drops his robe on the bed. He slides his jeans on and zips 'em up. The top button always gives him grief. Shaky fingers. Finally, the belt. This new belt has hooks. The old one had pairs of matching holes with corresponding tongs. Greg's tremors got so bad he could no longer line up the belt prongs and holes.

Washing and Shaving

Some things we barely think about are hard for tremblers. Washing hands and faces? Damned difficult. How come? Greg's trembling hands knock over the soft soap dispenser. Every time. In response, Greg reverted to bar soap in a big soap dish. It is hard to get the bar out of the dish. And Greg knocks the soap dish around the countertop. But he doesn't knock the soap dish over, breaking it. Eventually, Greg succeeds in getting the soap bar out of its dish.

Greg has an enormous goatee. It covers the bottom quarter of his face. With his goatee, he has less face to shave. Greg grew his goatee in self-defense. Back when he used scissors to keep it neat and trimmed, he stabbed himself. It did not take long for him to stop using the scissors.

Greg lathers up his face with the hot water and soap. Emma hops up on the counter. She rubs her face against his elbow. "Give me some room, Emma. You can't help me chip away at these whiskers. One day I may have to change to electric."

Buddy hops up beside Emma. The flowing hot water holds their interest. Both stare at the flowing water. Greg, conscientious about water use, turns the water off until he needs it again. Both cats stay in place, waiting for Greg to turn the water back on.

Greg picks up the razor. As carefully as possible, he bumps the blade against his skin. Bump, bump, bump. It is a wonder he doesn't cut himself. Much. Shaving takes a while. Five minutes, anyway. Satisfied, Greg pulls a face towel off the rack and dries.

"Just a couple more minutes, kitties. I have to brush my teeth." Emma sticks around. Buddy jumps down off the countertop and walks off. Greg picks up the toothpaste first. He holds the tube in his left hand. A shaking right hand goes for the cap. And misses. Greg lowers his left hand to the counter. The counter stabilizes the tube of toothpaste. It is enough. With the cap off, he reaches for his toothbrush.

Greg leans onto the countertop. Both forearms are on the sink's edge. His left hand holds the toothpaste. His right hand holds the brush. Slowly now! Ready? Aim. Squeeze.

Most of the time, the toothpaste ends up on his toothbrush. But, not always. Sometimes he misses completely. The toothpaste ends up in the sink. Today the toothpaste rests picture-perfect on Greg's toothbrush. One more step.

Greg shifts all his attention to his trembling right hand. He still must get the toothbrush into his mouth. Over time Greg learned to use his left hand to support his right. With his left hand facing up, he places his right wrist in his left palm. Now he is steady enough to get his toothbrush into his mouth.

Finally! Done.

Greg turns off the bathroom light. He gets a shirt out of the closet and puts it on. He finds the top button. Lining up buttons and holes is complicated. In the beginning, it wasn't that difficult. Sure, some days were harder than other days.

Even the time of day makes a difference. For Greg, about an hour after he gets up in the morning, his trembling is at its worst. That is right about now.

"You guys want to play? Buddy, where did you leave the paper? Did you leave it in your water dish again?"

Most cats won't play "fetch." Buddy and Emma are not like most cats. Greg tosses the crumpled ball of paper. Both cats leap on it, bat it around, kick it with hind feet, then bring it back near Greg. Although Buddy does like to dip the crumpled paper in his water dish, then dump it, unceremoniously, on the linoleum floor. Greg gets tired of the game before the cats do. He struggles with his buttons. The cats continue to play.

Breakfast

Well, that's enough. It is time for breakfast.

In the kitchen, Greg looks around. His tomato juice is still out on the counter. Using both hands, Greg lifts the sealed cup with the tomato juice in it to his mouth. His hands and arms bounce around, trembling wildly. He aims for the large straw. He sips it slowly, draining the red cup.

Tomato juice sucked through a straw is not much of a breakfast. "I think I will make some scrambled eggs," Greg thinks. He pulls a medium-sized mixing bowl out of a cabinet. He holds it as carefully as he can, so he won't drop it. Next, he selects the middle-sized frying pan and puts it on the stove. Greg moves from one cabinet to the next, gathering up oil, salt, pepper, and a fork. Last, he retrieves a carton of eggs from the fridge.

After opening the carton, Greg reaches for the first egg with his right hand. Picking things up is a challenge. His grip is not as "competent" as it once was. Many tremblers drop things. His left hand is over the top of his right hand. His trembling dampened, he picks up the egg and cracks it against the bowl's edge. The eggshell breaks into a half dozen pieces with extra shell pieces ending in the egg whites. He drops the broken eggshell into the garbage can and retrieves the eggshells from the mix. Greg takes a deep breath. "Whew." He breaks two more eggs.

Emma rubs herself against Greg's legs. "I can still shake the salt and pepper into my eggs," he tells Emma. He carefully picks up a fork. "Alright! I just gotta whip these eggs and cook em."

This could still be a good day.

Shopping

It is a shopping day. Greg doesn't shop every day. He shops just barely enough. "I hate that I have to ask for help," Greg thinks.

"You kitties seen my glasses?" Greg looks around for his glasses. "Where are they hiding this morning?" Buddy follows Greg, helpfully jumping up on the desk. The lens cleaning cloth is there. But no glasses. "How about on the nightstand, Buddy?" A quick look through the bedroom door and he scratches the nightstand off his mental list of possible places. "When did I have them last? Last night? Where might they be? There aren't that many options," he quizzes himself.

"Well, my glasses are either in the kitchen or the bathroom." As Greg is closest to the bathroom, he heads there first. "What do you know? There they are, right where I left them."

Greg picks up his glasses and uses both hands to put them on. He pads to the living room. Near his computer, he spots his lens cleaning cloths. Greg uses two. He carefully picks up the first cloth and places it in his left palm. He awkwardly lifts his glasses off his nose. Using his right hand, Greg guides the glasses until they rest between his left index finger and thumb. He cups the left lens between his fingers and the palm of his left hand. The side of the lens closest to his palm presses against the lens cloth.

Without a word, he picks up the other cloth in his right hand. Although both hands tremble, Greg knows he can line up the polishing cloth and lens. He polishes the right lens first with the other cloth. With one lens cleaned and shiny, he rotates the glasses, so a different lens is exposed. His trembling fingers line up on the second lens. In short order, Greg cleans and shines the second lens.

"I am going shopping. Do you guys want anything?"

Emma stares at Greg. Buddy's ears flick a couple of times.

"How about some tasty cat food? You are about out of cans."

Greg quickly takes inventory. Soup. Bagged cat food. Milk. Juice? Tomato? Apple? Cranberry? And maybe some hamburger. He knows he is kidding himself. When he gets to the store, he will walk down every aisle. He will find lots of things he didn't think of until the cart is half full.

It is a small town. Most everyone knows Greg. Greg knows most everyone. He starts in one aisle near the outside edge of the store. Most things are easy. Bread. Apples. Peaches. Easy. Lettuce. That is a little harder because it must slide into one of those flimsy, small, plastic bags. Up one aisle. Down the next.

Greg stops in front of the soups. Uh-oh. Every can is snuggled up to the ones beside it. He scans shelf after shelf after shelf. The soups form a solid, impenetrable tin wall. The soup cans stand steady as if they are an ancient Greek phalanx ready to defend themselves from attack. The defending soup cans stand twenty wide and five rows deep. Greg will win the Battle of the Soups. The costs will be high on both sides. His trembling hands will knock some cans off the shelf. Other cans will tumble backward toward the wall.

While Greg ponders his strategy, a woman walks into his view. Greg knows her. She is the store's customer service rep.

"Need some help, Greg?"

"Yes, Ma'am," he exclaims to the CSR!

Greg's reinforcement has tipped the Battle of the Soups in his favor. She has helped him before. And she will help him again. Greg chats and points out the half dozen soups he would like to buy. The customer service representative is happy to help. She remembers past experiences where cans ended up on the floor. This is the better option.

"Can I help you with anything else, Greg?"

"Do you have time to help me with some cat food? I need a half-dozen cans and one bag."

"Sure!" The cat food is two aisles over.

While they walk, she asks, "how are you doing?" Greg smiles broadly, "I am fine, thank you. How are you today?"

They chat back and forth. The CSR, the customer service representative, knows his story. Or she knows some of his stories. She has seen firsthand how he trembles. She knows Greg has trouble getting cans of food off her shelves. He tries hard not to, but he almost always knocks cans off shelves.

Almost always.

The customer service representative knows she has other customers who have tremors. Greg's are the worst.

"Here we are. Could you please get me a couple of cans of grilled chicken, maybe two cans of salmon, and three of those pates?"

"Sure, Greg. Anything else?"

"Yup. One small bag of Friskies. Thanks."

Greg smiles. He hates it when he must ask for help. Last week he was embarrassed when he asked another shopper for help. She looked at his trembling hands, then hurried on her way. Most people don't know what tremors are. We have more than three hundred million souls in the United States. About ten million have essential tremor. Many who have them live with their trembling limbs, just as Greg did. Most people who have ET don't know it is a medical condition.

Greg knows.

"Could you help me with one more thing?"

The CSR nods. "Glad to."

"I need a pound of hamburger. Last time I put my fingers right through the package," Greg explained.

"Let's go pick out the one you want."

Shopping? Done.

Gasoline

It was not too bad this time. "Time to fill-up and check the mail on my way home," Greg thinks as he drives. He stops at the Exxon station, where Sue works. Newport is a small town. It only takes him a couple of minutes to get there.

Greg pulls his truck up to one of the pumps, shuts off his engine, and hops out. His vehicle came with a locking gas cap. To get the cap off, he lines up the key with the keyhole. There isn't enough space to use one hand to guide his fingers. Instead, Greg holds the key in his right hand, then places his right hand and wrist into his left hand. With his left thumb in his right palm and his fingers curling around his right wrist, he has the stability he needs. He moves his hands up and down as well as from side to side as he aligns the key with the keyhole. On each attempt, Greg has a good chance of getting the key into the keyhole. Occasionally, he succeeds on his first try. But not this day.

Once. Twice. Three times. Nope. Four tries. The fifth time's a charm. Good. Pumping the gas is easy compared to getting the cap off.

It's time to pay. Greg heads inside to pay. It is easier.

At the grocery store, he used his debit card to pay for his groceries. Most of the check-out clerks know Greg needs help with his card.

"Would you mind," he asks the clerk handing her his debit card? After she easily inserts the card into the reader, Greg uses the thumb and second finger of his right hand to hold onto the card reader. He presses the PIN with his index finger.

"Can I ask you a question?" the clerk asks Greg.

"Sure."

"Are you okay? You are shaking."

"It is called ET, essential tremor. It is not contagious. It is a conversation starter." Greg smiles. "I tremble, mostly in my hands and arms. You can't see them, but I also have the same tremors in my chest and upper back. I even get them in my legs."

"I am so sorry!"

"Lots of people have tremors. You probably know others. Most tremors aren't so obvious as mine. Would you like to know more? My brother has it too. He has a website where he writes articles about essential tremor. Here is a card with his website on it."

"Always Heading North? What a strange name. Thanks, I will look," the check-out clerk said.

"Who knows what my brother was thinking? Anyway, we are writing my story, and he is posting about it there," Greg continues.

Here, at the gas station, Greg hands the register clerk a small wad of bills. He lets the clerk count out the right amount. Handling paper money is beyond Greg's ability.

He heads home. After he puts away the groceries, he plays with Emma and Buddy for a few minutes. And just like that, it is time for lunch.

Lunchtime

"Peanut butter and jelly today? Or bologna and cheese?" Greg pulls a couple of slices of bread out of the wrapper. He gets a knife out of the drawer, opens the refrigerator, and gathers up the Miracle Whip and mustard. He has made up his mind. He sets everything on the countertop. He returns to the fridge and selects a small plastic bottle of Coke. The bottle goes on the counter, too. Finally, he gets the packages of bologna and cheese.

Greg runs some warm water over his hands and wipes them dry on the dishtowel. He peels off a slice of bologna and places it on the leftmost piece of bread. The cheese is next. His trembling fingers do the best he can to slice off two lovely, thick pieces of cheese. After just a couple of tries, Greg succeeds. He lays the cheese on top of the bologna.

He grips the Miracle Whip jar with his right hand. He uses his left hand to unscrew the cap. So far, so good. Greg uses his left hand now to hold the container. His wildly trembling right hand grips the knife. He has a good sense of humor. He grins, knows what is coming. He tries to keep the amount of spread on the blade to the smallest possible amount. The tip of the knife bounces wildly. The first glob to break loose lands right in the middle of the bread. What good luck! "Ha," Greg exclaims!

The second glob lands on the counter. "Darn!"

Another scoop. This time Greg gets Miracle Whip all over his fingers. It happens every time. But he persists. The Miracle Whip finally gets spread. The dab of mustard magically finds its way onto his sandwich. And cleanup is not that hard either. "I wonder if the squeezable Miracle Whip jars are better?" Greg ponders.

One more thing about lunch. Eating is always a contest. Drinking sucks! Greg fashioned a technique for how not to spill his Coke. It goes something like this. First, hold the bottle and get the cap off. Second, hold the bottle with both hands. The container remains firmly on the countertop. He slowly lowers his mouth to near the top of the bottle. With some effort, he lines up his mouth with the bottle top. Once the container is in his mouth, Greg lifts the bottle and drinks.

Living with essential tremor takes patience and effort. Once tremors become a part of one's life, every simple task needs a new look. Every simple task becomes difficult. Or messy. Some tasks become impossible. The luckiest people have someone who can help them with impossible tasks.

Greg's thoughts turn to Sue. "Thank goodness for Sue."

He smiles. Sue helps a lot!

With essential tremor, some days are worse than others. So far, this day has been about in the middle. Greg trembles worst in the morning. Sometimes he has trouble breathing when he first wakes up. In addition to tremors, he also has COPD, a breathing disorder.

"I have trouble holding the inhaler still. It is hard to get the cap off the darned thing. Once the cap is off, I steady my right hand with my left hand. Then I line up the distributor with my mouth. It is harder than it sounds."[1]

Every trembler needs help from time to time. Essential tremor never get "better" without intervention. At the beginning of our lifelong journey, our problems may be small, evenly matched to the help we receive from those who love us. At first, we need help with simple things like buttoning a button or filling out a form. We can make adjustments in how we approach our tasks. For easy cases, like Steven's, simple devices like "stiff" mechanical keyboards and programmable mice, let him do most of his daily tasks without help. But handwriting is another matter. Writing a check to pay for a service is impossible for Steven. Someone else has to write checks.

Harder cases, like Greg's, can wear down a partner, whether a spouse, parent or close friend. We are meant to be mostly self-sufficient. Even as tremblers we must look for ways to do things for ourselves whenever we can. Be vocal in commercial settings. Ask for help and ask for alternatives. As an example, Steven always asked for the option to fill out forms online. At first, almost no one offered the opportunity. Now, most specialty clinics will send a link to a patient portal. Many banks provide bill-paying services entirely online. We must do as much for ourselves as we can.

Parents of tremblers will have to train their children to be self-sufficient as much as possible. This can be hard. Tough love always is. Children may take the easy way and let parents do things for them instead of finding new ways to do something for themselves. Be patient. Help your children discover the things they can do.

Greg and Sue discovered Greg's tremors together. Greg's life held minor inconveniences in the beginning. Fine motor skills, working with our hands, are usually the first skills to disappear. Greg lost the ability to tie fishing flies and to prepare a line with a hook and bait for fishing. Less obviously, Greg's handwriting became unreadable. When it came time to choose, Greg's employer laid him off in a downturn. No more fishing. No more job.

In the beginning, Sue simply did what was necessary. She didn't say much. She saw Greg's problems and helped solve them. Tremblers spill things. Sue bought large cups with lids and straw holes. Sue helped Greg simplify and adjust.

In the hardest cases, the Trembler may need far more help than a spouse, parent, or close friend can give. On some days, some tremblers cannot feed themselves. Personal hygiene is tough for both tremblers and helpers. When possible, hire some additional help. We have an industry built around giving extra support to the aged and infirm.

Chapter Eight: Essential Tremor Is Real

"Why me? What did I do? Why do I tremble? What can I do about it?" Greg's questions are the right questions. Why him? How did it begin? What did he do wrong? For Greg, the most crucial issue is what can he do about his tremors?

His questions have no satisfying answers. Not today.

Doctors are slow to learn about tremors. Essential tremor, or ET, is a movement disorder. The best current guess is about ten million Americans have it.[1] Tremors don't kill anybody. Not directly anyway. When you talk to enough people with ET, you will find many are embarrassed, anxious, and stressed. Almost everyone who has it notices their loss of fine motor skills. Using small screwdrivers or knives or even writing pens, become difficult. Things we once found easy become hard to do.

People new to tremors want to know what to expect. They want to know how essential tremor will progress. Most tremblers, in the beginning, are only vaguely aware something is not quite right. One of the authors believes ET is the result of damage that slowly accumulates in our brains. The parts of our brain that coordinate our movements lose their ability to synchronize opposing muscle pairs. At some point, we recognize our trembling. And we "suddenly" realize, we have ET. Perhaps, for a long time, years, the damage will continue to accumulate. Our tremors may appear to be about the same. We reach another awareness threshold. Over time we may move from mild shaking to wild shaking and from occasional shaking to near-continuous shaking.

ET affects everything. Men and women with ET complain about other serious problems. Greg has some but not others. No one knows if ET causes the other issues. Or vice versa. Maybe all the problems share a common foundation.

What we do know is people with tremors complain about these other things. At the top of the list are stress, anxiety, tinnitus, and sleep disorders. Many also complain about depression, dizziness, isolation, embarrassment, and stammering.

Essential tremor usually start "small."

"I just have the shakes."

"I don't know why I keep dropping my pen. I guess I am just clumsy."

"Just half a cup. Sometimes I spill it."

"I can't seem to hit the head of the screw today. I need a better screwdriver."

"I can't bait my hook today."

"I am just high strung."

"I just have bad handwriting."

We don't see our doctor. We don't know what our complaint is. Not right away, anyway. Eventually, our symptoms, hands, and arms that tremble as we do things grow more noticeable. People may ask why we shake. At some point, we know we need to see our doctor.

Most doctors don't know about ET either. Because doctors are generally unaware, we must prepare ourselves before we see our doctor. There are things we can and should do before we set up an appointment. As we develop our plans, some questions will become apparent. Other issues might not be as obvious. Movement disorder and Essential Tremor websites, medical websites, and Facebook groups all contain items like the ones we ask. These questions are not original to the authors.

If we believe we may have a movement disorder like essential tremor we can ask ourselves some clarifying questions:

What are my symptoms?

1) What parts of my body are involved? Beginning at the top of my head and working my way down to my feet, I consider the following:

- Head. Does my head nod up and down (yes-yes) or move from side to side (no-no)?
- Face. Do any parts of my face twitch? Some people report eyelids, jaws, and lip twitches.
- Voice. Does my voice quiver?
- Neck. Does my neck quiver or twitch?
- Shoulders, upper back, and upper chest. In some people, the trembling is perceptible. Others must be still to notice.
- Arms. Do parts of my arms twitch or tremble?
- Hands. Do my hands or fingers shake?
- Trunk. Do any parts of my abdomen or back twitch, quiver, tremble or shake?
- Legs. Do any parts of my legs tremble or twitch?
- Feet. Do my feet twitch or tremble?

- Do I have balance problems?

2) For the parts of my body that shake, tremble or twitch, think about when it happens.

- Do I tremble when I am at rest?
- Does my trembling begin with purposeful movements or holding things against gravity?
- Does drinking increases my trembling? Many people first notice their trembling while holding a cup or glass.
- Does eating increase my trembling? Do things that can fall off a fork or spoon fall off?
- Do my hands tremble when I am writing?

3) When do I notice trembling?

- Do I tremble when I first wake up in the morning?
- Does my trembling increase throughout the day?
- Is it worst late in the day?
- Do I tremble occasionally?
- Do I tremble all the time?

4) How severe are my symptoms?

- Mild?
- Severe?
- Do my symptoms vary?

5) What makes my symptoms worse? Here are a few factors to think about:

- Anxiety,
- Caffeine (coffee, tea, colas),
- Fatigue,

- Hunger, smoking, stress,
- Extreme temperatures (freezing and sweltering),
- Alcohol (a little may reduce tremors).

Other Factors

1) What other medical problems do I have?

2) What other human issues do I have?

- Am I anxious, stressed, or depressed?
- Am I sleeping well?
- Do I have tinnitus?

3) What medications and over the counter supplements am I taking?

As a useful reminder and to save time in the doctor's office, consider keeping a text file with the prescription medications you take, the doses, and when you take them. Leave a few spaces then continue with any dietary supplements you take, their dosages, and when you take them. The night before your appointment, update the file and print a copy for your doctor to put in your medical record.

4) What is my medical history?

- Do I have any allergies or reactions to medications?
- Have I had any surgeries?

5) What is my general health?

6) What is my dental health?

Questions for my doctor

1) Experience and qualifications

- How long have you been practicing medicine (if it is a new doctor)?
- Have you treated anyone else with a movement disorder like essential tremor?

2) Diagnosis

- What do I have? What is this disease, condition, or disorder? Do I have essential tremor? How do you know? Are there things I can do or stop doing to reduce my symptoms?
- How serious is it? How will it affect my home, social, and work lives? Can others get this from me? Should I have safety concerns?
- How did I get it, or what caused it? Is there more than one disease, condition, or disorder that could cause my symptoms?
- Should I have any lab tests? What will the test results tell me? Will the tests confirm I have something? Or will they refute something?
- How safe and accurate are the tests?
- Will I need follow-up visits? If so, how frequently?
- What are the short term and long-term outlooks for me? Will I return to normal?

3) Treatment

- What treatment is most common for my condition?
- What are my treatment options?
- What is the least amount of treatment?
- What is the most significant amount of treatment?
- How are others with my symptoms and condition treated?

- What do you recommend?
- What will happen if I do not treat this?
- What happens if I delay treatment?
- What medicines will you prescribe?
    - What are the most likely side effects?
    - What should I do if I have side effects?
    - What are the benefits?
    - What are the risks?
    - How will I know if the medicines are working?
    - Is there anything I should avoid doing during treatment?
- Will the new medicines interact with anything I am currently taking?
- What impact will my new medicines have on my gut biome?
- How will treatment affect my job or lifestyle?
- How much will it cost to treat my condition?

4) What do I expect from my doctor?

- Why am I seeing my doctor?
- What do I expect to happen as a result of seeing my doctor?
- Is my doctor listed on any of the doctor rating sites? Here are two locations: Healthgrades and Zocdocs.

Ask questions. Get answers. Then you will begin to understand your disorder and what you can do about it.

Chapter Nine: Essential Tremor Plus Nine

In this chapter, we will discuss movement disorders plus nine more things people who have essential tremor also tend to have.

- What is a movement disorder?
- What are the six other big things we may also have?
- What are the three other minor things we may also have?

Let's begin with the basics.

What is a Movement Disorder?

As one human being with a movement disorder to another, a movement disorder is an unwanted movement we have little control over. We tremble when we are not afraid. If we shake at rest, we may have one kind of movement disorder. If we tremble when we are holding a posture against gravity, we may have another type of movement disorder.

Medical websites like Medline Plus, a government website, say there are at least six major movement disorders.[1] We rewrote most of their awkward sentences. Here is their alphabetized list:

- Ataxia, the loss of muscle coordination.
- Dystonia, in which your muscles twist and move repetitively. The movements can be painful.

- Huntington's disease, in which nerve cells in parts of our brains, that help control voluntary movements waste away.
- Parkinson's disease causes tremors, slowness of movement, and trouble walking. It gets worse over time.
- Tourette syndrome causes people to make sudden twitches, movements, or sounds (tics).
- Tremor and essential tremor causes involuntary trembling or shaking movements. The movements may be in one or more parts of your body.

What causes movement disorders?

Doctors give movement disorders and their underlying mechanisms, many fancy names. We found about a dozen different, complicated medical names for the most common movement disorders. Each describes a combination of muscles, nerves, and actions within our spinal cord and brains where one or more things have gone wrong. For now, we can let our doctors worry about naming things. In general, we have movement disorders because something has gone wrong with our nervous systems, including our brains, spinal columns, and nerves.

How Do Movement Disorders Begin?

It is different for each of us.

Steven, a US Army Major, trembled. He dropped ink pens. Something wasn't right. His fingers trembled, although he wasn't nervous. His once excellent note-taking handwriting was no longer crisp and clear. For Steven, it started with his hands.

Steven is right-handed. When he dropped things, they fell from his right hand. He held his coffee cup in his right hand. Steven explained, "As I held my cup, I could see the coffee moving back and forth, side to side. I could tell my hand was shaking. Others noticed it too. At first, it did not happen all the time. But the trembling became more frequent. Sometimes I spilled my coffee. The people I worked with commented. I started to hide my hands. So, I went to see my doctor."

Other Movement Disorder Experiences[2]

Emma's tremors had a different beginning. "Someone asked me at work, 'why is your head like a nodding dog'? I had felt stressed and 'on edge' for a while but couldn't put my finger on what was wrong. I got very upset at what he had said as I didn't understand it. I got so paranoid about it; I even started to video my movements to try to get perspective on what other people saw. It was an awfully difficult time."

Martine remembers "vibrating" at the young age of ten or eleven. At first, it was one hand. Then both hands. "My doctors said I was nervous, or I was too high strung, or they even told me it was high metabolism. Most people ignored my vibrating."

Nicola commented, "I was in my early 20s when my shaky hands become apparent. My mum joked it was because I drank too much. It wasn't until I was 37, I was diagnosed. My hands were getting worse. Obviously, my shaking wasn't alcohol related. And people at work had started to notice and comment on my shakes."

Michael recalled, "I was 5 or 6 when teachers noticed it. My parents took me to the doctor, who explained, 'he just grew too fast for his nervous system.' So that's what I told people for years. Then I learned that was nonsense. But it didn't change the fact that I shook, and I had to learn how to adapt. Luckily, I learned to laugh at the condition and myself. Otherwise, I never would have survived my school years."

Sheri told me, "My mom passed away in June 2011. Not long after that, I thought something was happening. I went to get a haircut, and I had like a little spasm in my neck, and my head twitched. I was 48. Mind you, I will see my first neurologist in June to know for sure. Mine is still mild. First, my hands, mostly when writing, then my head. Most recently, I feel internal tremors."

Mike relayed his story. "I was 18, it was my senior year in high school, 1985. I wanted to be a welder when I graduated, didn't know yet what field, just that I loved working with my hands, was very good at trigonometry, really enjoyed complex problem solving, that sort of thing, and I loved being outdoors.

A local pipeline welder let me work part-time for him and he began to teach me the basics. If you're unfamiliar with welders or construction workers in general, suffice it to say that there isn't any coddling happening on the jobsite. I had no clue at this point that I had essential tremor. I hadn't even noticed myself shaking-but when I started welding it didn't take long for me to earn the nickname 'Shaky' – as in – 'Dang Shaky, I don't know how you're doing it but that bead looks okay to me'… or my favorite 'Settle down, Shaky - you're shaking harder than a dog trying to crap a peach seed!'"

Greg, the author, first noticed light tremors after a horrible car accident that left his right arm badly damaged. He had pins in his left hand. The car accident mangled his three leftmost fingers. Metal pins held his bones in place. On his return to the hospital to have the pins removed, he noticed a mild trembling for the first time. His notice rapidly passed. He gave it no further thought. Maybe the trembling was his body's way of dealing with having the pins pulled out. Greg's tremors had a slow, mild beginning. It took about two years before his tremors were visible both to himself and to others. Like most of us, Greg noticed the trembling but thought nothing of it. Over time he realized he was trembling more often. He had trouble doing more things. People he worked with begin to comment. Like most of us, Greg didn't realize he had a problem.

If you are reading this, you may be trembling as we were. You may think you have essential tremor or Parkinson's Disease or something else. Or you live with someone who shakes. You want to know more.[3]

Like other medical conditions, each trembler has her own symptoms and timelines. Steven's symptoms remained constant for almost a decade. Then his symptoms increased month by month until they reached another plateau. Greg's symptoms began gradually and increased gradually over two years. He too, has reached a plateau. Both authors notice day to day changes with some days having less trembling and other days having far more. We each experience our own timelines.

Essential tremor as a problem is like every other human problem. We must cope with our challenges as they come. Some things we like to do may be taken away from us. For some of us writing is no longer possible. And some of us need mechanical keyboards and programmable mice so we can continue using our computers. We can and must find things we enjoy doing. Greg started gardening or as he put it, "going outside and pushing dirt around."

The authors have a short wish list for assistive devices you can find in chapter seventeen.

What is Essential Tremor?

What do we know today? We have a definition of sorts. Essential tremor is a movement disorder. ET is a "neurological condition that most commonly causes a rhythmic trembling of the hands while performing a task..."[4] The motions are uncontrollable, involuntary. The shaking or trembling is rhythmic.

What Causes Essential Tremor?

We don't know what causes essential tremor. But doctors have some ideas. Most websites discuss abnormal brain activity. "One theory suggests that your cerebellum and other parts of your brain are not communicating correctly. The cerebellum controls muscle coordination."[5] Another popular theory claims the abnormal brain activity originates in the thalamus. The thalamus plays a significant role in coordination and controlling muscle activities. Medline Plus lists a few probable causes. They include genetics, infections, metabolic disorders, damage to our brains, spinal cord, or peripheral nerves, metabolic disorders, stroke, and vascular diseases, and toxins.[6]

Doctors and researchers do not believe ET is part of aging. We do not automatically get essential tremor as we age. If we have essential tremor, our symptoms increase as we age. Each of us can attest to that. As we age, our occasional tremors may become a constant companion.

Tremors can affect anyone at any age. The authors have secondhand knowledge of children as young as six who have essential tremor. Most of the people who have it first recognize that something is wrong during their 40s to 50s. It becomes more common as we age. One medical website claims that it is common in people over age 65 with as many as four million affected.[7]

Okay. We have it. How did we get it? There are two significant ways to get it. Parents pass essential tremor to their children genetically. About half of the known cases have a known genetic origin. A child born to a parent with essential tremor has a 50% chance of having it too.

It also occurs when no parent is known to have had essential tremor.

Some factors do not cause essential tremor but may play a role. Here are some examples:

- Thyroid problems.
- Alcohol abuse. A small amount of alcohol can reduce tremors. A large amount can increase tremor amplitude.
- Some prescription drugs may make essential tremor worse.
- A stroke may make the symptoms worse.

One of the authors, Steven, believes essential tremor is the result of a combination of genetics, epigenetics, and body-wide inflammation. There is a growing body of evidence that suggests ET is a common neurodegenerative disorder. Parkinson's disease, multiple sclerosis, Alzheimer's disease, and depression all correlate with inflammation.[8]

Chapter Ten: Stress

Besides tremors, people with ET commonly report other issues. In an informal survey of a half dozen popular Facebook support groups, the authors discovered six major additional problems routinely reported by people with essential tremor.[1] Not everyone experiences all six. Many people experience two or more. Here are the top six additional problems:

- Stress
- Anxiety
- Tinnitus
- Sleep disorders
- Depression
- Dizziness

There were three other complaints we classified as minor complaints. These complaints are not less worrisome. They drew fewer comments. Here are the three additional claims:

- Stammering
- Embarrassment
- Isolation

In addition to coping with a movement disorder like essential tremor, it is also necessary to deal with the added problems.

Let's begin with stress.

The dictionary defines stress as a form of mental tension, which builds up in people when they are facing adverse situations. Robert Sapolsky, Ph.D., tells stories about good stress and bad stress. If, as you get out of your car after driving home from work unexpectedly find yourself face to face with a lion, you run! That is good stress.

Your body stops doing everything that can be put off to face the immediate, life, and death situation. Your heart and breathing rates increase. Your body dumps as much sugar into your bloodstream as possible—energy courses through your big muscles. Being chased by a lion is a single event. One way or another, the game is quickly resolved. Our stress rapidly rises. Then it returns to normal. If we survive, we have a great story to tell.

But we can also turn on stress with just a thought or an emotion. When we do, the same things happen in our bodies as when we came face to face with the lion. When we do it too often, it becomes bad stress. It becomes chronic. It wears us out. Unresolved stress leads to other serious problems.[2] Chronic stress causes three of the issues frequently reported by others with essential tremor. Anxiety, sleep disorders, and depression can all result from repeated, unresolved stress. Here is an alphabetized list, derived from ten books we read on stress, and one Great Courses series:

- Anxiety
- Breathing changes
- Cancer (possibly)
- Digestive system problems
- Increased heart rate and blood pressure
- Immune system compromise
- Headaches
- Liver problems
- Sleep disorders

Chronic stress drains our body's resources. Its effects accumulate. We should do something about bad stress.

Why do people with tremors experience stress? First, stress is part of the human condition. From time to time, everyone experiences stress. Robert Sapolsky described the things that cause stress or stressors this way. A stressor is anything that knocks us off balance. A stressor is also anything that makes us think we are about to be knocked off balance. It can be a real thing, or it can be a thought, our response to a situation, real, imagined, or re-lived.

Real or imagined. Is it any wonder we have so much stress in our lives?

What can people with essential tremor (ET) do to cope with stress? First, we can recognize the problem. We can accept that we must find ways to deal with the stress we experience. We can begin with the simplest things. If we divide stressors into major groupings, we can tackle them, one group, at a time. Let's create an alphabetized list. Why? We like alphabetized lists. Here is ours wholly influenced by the books we have read and websites we visited:

- Biogenic
- Physical (activities and conditions)
- Psychosocial

Let's begin with biogenic. Tina Taylor, in her book *Stress Effects*, identifies food classes, medicines, and things we ingest, inhale or inject as biogenic stressors.[3] Other authors have similar lists. Knowing and changing the food classes we eat can be useful for reducing stress. For example, a shift toward a vegetarian diet reduces biogenic stress. Dr. David

Perlmutter, in his book *Grain Brain*, makes the case that our brains thrive on healthy fats and healthy cholesterol. Sugars and carbohydrates damage our brains.[4]

Other food classes, or choices, can be harmful. Processed foods, including many fast foods, and many commercial baked foods are loaded with simple sugars and trans-fatty acids. Let's take sugars. Too much sugar, whether directly consumed or in the form of carbohydrates, is linked to anxiety, cancer, depression, dementia, multiple sclerosis, Parkinson's, and Alzheimer's disease, heart disease, and strokes.

The undesirable foods listed above contain emulsifiers. Because oil and water don't mix without help, we add food emulsifiers. Food emulsifiers help water and oils mix, prevent separation, and create a smooth texture. Emulsifiers also appear to cause a low level of inflammation. It is too early to say with certainty, but emulsifiers may change our gut biome. Eating processed foods can lead to digestive problems and something horrible called leaky gut.

We don't have to cut them out, but we can reduce our exposure to them to cope with bad stress.

Some medicines add to our stress as a side effect. They can also change our gut biome.[5] In the last few years, the amount we have learned about our gut, our stomach, small intestines, and our large intestines has grown enormously. While we don't entirely understand, it is becoming clear that a healthy gut biome is essential to health. So, make a list of your medicines, then search the Internet to see what impacts your medications may have on your gut biome. Discuss what you find with your doctor.

We can eat foods to improve the health and diversity of bacteria that live in our gut. We can eat more pre-biotic foods. These support the enormous numbers of bacteria we need for healthy living. We can also eat more probiotic foods. These probiotic foods help build the right sorts of bacteria colonies. As in every case, decide what you want to do, then discuss it with your doctor. Some pre and probiotics may have side effects.

The third large area is the things we ingest, inhale, or inject. Caffeine, we regret to report, is on the list of biogenic stressors. So is nicotine. Tina Taylor, in *Stress Effects*, offers a long list. Here is a sample: amphetamine and methamphetamine, caffeine, Gingko Biloba, Ginseng, nicotine, phenylpropanolamine, theobromine, theophylline, and yohimbine.[6]

Whew! We admit we do not know what most of them are. Check labels of the things in your life. If you spot one look it up, see if it is essential or optional. Then decide to keep it, reduce it, or discard it to cope with stress.

The next great area is physical, neatly divided into activities and conditions. We will just hit the top couple as a sampler: illness, pain, sleep deprivation, hunger or food deprivation, and sexual performance. Tina Taylor offers a much longer list in her book.[7]

The psychosocial stressors make up the third area. These fall into two groups, challenges and the things we fear. We feel stress because we view them as a threat. Challenges involve something new, unexpected, or novel. We cannot predict the outcome. Two other things are essential for a challenge to cause bad stress. We do not have control, and our egos or personalities are threatened.

The list of things to be feared is long and varied. We each have our list of fears. Here are a few of the more popular fears, given as examples: loss of our job, inability to manage our finances (too much month at the end of the money), and our schedules (way more things to do than there is time left to do them).[8]

How do we cope with bad stress? We have some general thoughts derived almost entirely from the books we read (and that one Great Courses course).

Some of these ideas may sound notably "New Age-ish." For example, change what you can change. Accept the things that cannot be changed. Reinhold Niebuhr wrote something he called "The Prayer." It went like this.

"Father, give us courage to change what must be altered, serenity to accept what cannot be helped, and the insight to know the one from the other."

Someone altered the words somewhat to give us this:

"God grant me the serenity to accept the things I cannot change,

Courage to change the things I can,

And the wisdom to know the difference."

Change what can be changed. Accept what cannot be changed.

One New Age thought leads to another. The Serenity Prayer led me to remember Max Ehrmann's Desiderata. Although copyright prevents me from publishing it all, a simple web search will pull it up for you.

"Go placidly amid the noise and haste,

and remember what peace there may be in silence.

As far as possible without surrender

be on good terms with all persons.

Speak your truth quietly and clearly;

and listen to others,

even the dull and the ignorant;

they too have their story."[9]

Another general idea for coping with bad stress is to keep a journal. Essential tremor may have ruined our handwriting. But it is possible to keep an electronic journal. Speech to text software is inexpensive. Learning to use speech to text does take effort. We must remember to speak in our punctuation. Those commas, periods, question marks, and exclamation points are not going to write themselves!

Keeping a journal lets us document our days and weeks. We can be thoughtful and reflective as we capture what caused our stress. For essential tremor, we may be embarrassed when we must do things in public. We may be frustrated because we knock things over or find we can no longer do simple tasks like buttoning our shirts or tying our shoes.

From time to time, we can look back through our journal entries to help us identify our unique stressors. Some everyday stressors include nearby neighbors, barking dogs, other loose, roaming pets, perhaps traffic, or a boss.

Once we have a list, we can begin to understand what we do when we are stressed. Many of us eat, drink, or smoke. Maybe we scratch. Perhaps we become agitated. So, make your list. Next, review your list. Decide, one by one, which stress habits you want to change. Some stress habits, such as eating, drinking, or smoking, may be tough to change or end. Still, it is worth exploring to see if there is a healthier alternative. Instead of reaching for that candy bar, we can substitute some raw nuts or berries instead. Consider that stress often leads to poor diets. We make poor choices. Our digestive system may be out of balance, so nutrients are not absorbed as well. Chronic stress depletes some essential nutrients.

Melissa Hartwig and Dr. David Perlmutter recommend substantial dietary changes designed to improve one's whole health. A side benefit may include stress reduction.

Sometimes the stressors are complicated. Is it my job or my boss? What if it is my spouse? Keeping a stress diary can help establish where the stress originates. Be specific. Write down the date and time.

- What happened?
- What was said?
- Who said it?
- Who was involved?
- Was it hard to breathe?
- Did your stomach or head hurt?

- Were there other physical sensations?
- Were you nervous or angry or frustrated?

Think it through. Rate your stress for this event. Use a scale that works for you. Some people use a range of one to five where one is unremarkably low, but noticeable stress. And five is unbearable stress.

If my stress is due to my job or boss, is it due to unrealistic expectations?

- Is it my work schedule?
- Would a vacation help solve it?
- Should I consider a job change?
- Should I think of a career change?
- Is there a reasonable way to change my current condition?

If it is due to noisy neighbors, would a privacy fence help?

Sometimes it helps to talk to a friend.

Growing up, we often heard that laughter is the best medicine. When we laugh, we release endorphins. Endorphins make us feel good. What helps you laugh? Find a way to include laughter in your daily routine. Many people stumble into unhelpful strategies that make matters worse.

- We avoid confronting the stressors.
- We make excuses.
- We stop doing activities.
- We may become isolated or even depressed.

Or we pick up addictive habits. Comfort foods loaded with sugars, unhealthy fats, or caffeine, or alcohols make us feel better. But only briefly. Or we smoke.

We can behave differently. Greg discovered that heading out to his backyard garden helps. Under stress, he moves some dirt around. Things seem better.

We can make long-term lifestyle changes. Some are easy. We can learn how to breathe better. Loris Vitry, in his book *Breathe Like a Master*, explains how breathing like a master calms our body and our mind. Loris claims breathing is the basis for physical and mental health. His technique, called intermittent breathing, is simple to practice. Breathe only through the nose. Breathe in slowly and naturally. Breathe out slowly and naturally. Pause naturally. Practice observantly for twenty minutes.[10]

We can exercise. Get up! We sit too much. Stand up. Walk around. Remain in motion. Lift light to moderate weights. Spend time outside. There are many exercise options. In addition to walking, we can do aerobics four times per week. We can learn and practice Tai Chi or yoga. Or other flexibility exercises. Exercises reduce stress levels. It is effective against anxiety and depression.

Other lifestyle changes range from simple like chew gum, spend time in the sun, and start a new hobby. Other lifestyle changes are a little harder. We can learn how to be grateful. Make a list of the positive things in your life, and read it frequently. Learn to eat well. Learn to sleep well. Learn that it is okay to say, "No." Some lifestyle changes may be especially hard. Let people go who routinely cause stress.

Terminate relationships, if possible. If it is not possible, then limit your contact with stress-inducing people.

Lower the drama.[11] We don't have to fight every battle nor right every wrong. An insightful person long ago said, "When things go wrong, don't go with them."[12] And learn from mistakes, both your own and others.

Turn off the TV news. Turn off or limit talk radio. Find alternative routes to work. Remember, we each, alone, are responsible for our happiness and well-being.

Hardest of all is to build a life around one's values. Near the end of the last century, Hyrum Smith wrote a fascinating book called *The 10 Natural Laws of Successful Time and Life Management*. His ten laws show how we can identify our real values, then build a life around our values.

In addition to lifestyle changes, consider trying and mastering relaxation techniques. There are many. Steven's favorites are the Five Ms. Massage. Meditation. Mindfulness. Muscle relaxation. And Moderate exercise. There are many inexpensive books available to choose from and explore each "M."

We should learn and practice some relaxation techniques we can use in the moment of stress. Some are listed above. Intermittent breathing. Learn to relax our faces and smile. Learn to counter teeth grinding. William Whitman, in his book *Playful Stress Reducing Shortcuts*, speaks of owl eyes and owl ears. Stress leads to tunnel vision. When we train our peripheral vision, we reduce our stress. When we listen with owl ears, we focus on the sounds emerging from a field of stillness. We calm our minds.[13]

Chapter Eleven: Anxiety

Second to stress people with essential tremor experience anxiety.

David Green, in his book *Anxiety Management and Stress Relief*, discusses how stress, unsuccessfully managed, can lead to anxiety and even depression. But what is anxiety? After reading seven books and skimming a dozen websites, it is unclear what it is. Every book describes anxiety symptoms. One site says it is a worry or fear that does not go away. That is simple enough. But it is not satisfying. Should we add that the worry, concern, or fear is unreasonable? After all, if our fears or worries are reasonable, is it anxiety? Dunno.

Let's set that aside. Everyone provided lists of symptoms. Every book. Every author. Every website. Your fearless authors pulled together a list we made from everyone else's lists. We like lists. And we love alphabetized lists. Here is ours:

- Aches or tensions in the muscles (with no other explanation)
- A chronic feeling of unease
- Clammy palms
- Dizziness or feeling light-headed
- Dry mouth
- Excessive sweating
- Exhaustion or fatigue
- Heart racing – irregular or fast heartbeat
- Panic attacks
- Shortness of breath
- Sleep disorders (with no other explanation)

- Sudden fears
- Trembling or shaking

With a list, this long, is it any wonder researchers claim at least 19 million Americans are affected by anxiety? Just look at that list. No one will have all the symptoms. But we all experience one or more of these symptoms from time to time. When do occasional symptoms become a problem?

Rose Heather, in her book, *7 Top Anxiety Management Techniques*, provides clues. This author took Rose's clues and converted them into, you guessed it, an alphabetized word group. We call it dread, fear, nervousness, and worry. We even made an acronym: Dread | Fear | Nervousness | Worry (DFNW).[1]

Sometimes DFNW is normal. We are threatened. We are in danger. We really should prepare to run or fight. But most of the time it is just traffic. Or noise. Or neighbors. Or barking dogs. Or our boss. Or, well, you get the point, but our bodies don't.

How do we deal with it? How do we deal with anxieties that, at times, overwhelm us? Rose Heather describes two significant options, treatments, and techniques.

Treatments.

Treatments include evidence-based medicine, therapy, and complementary and alternative options. Of the three, seeing a doctor is a good option for most people. Your doctor can help you understand your symptoms and can prescribe medicines for you. Drugs can help quickly. However, all drugs have side effects. Some people see the side effects as more harmful than the problem itself. Nor does medication identify and help you manage the underlying problem. Still, seeing your doctor is an excellent place to start.

Another choice many people make is therapy. Therapy comes in a variety of packages. A therapist can help you choose one or some combination of several therapy options. In general, any treatment helps you to understand why you are anxious. And in general, all therapies use different methods to help you change your thinking and your response to anxieties. Some ask you to keep a journal. Some expose you to whatever it is that makes you anxious while keeping you in a safe environment. It is unclear how that works if your problem is your boss. Some help you to accept your condition and learn how to cope. No therapy works for everybody, but each treatment works for some people.

Many people begin with complementary and alternative methods for managing or controlling anxieties. Like the other choices, all these methods work for some people. None of them work for all people. They include acupuncture, herbal remedies like teas, relaxation techniques, and yoga.[2] While not explicitly mentioned, the authors include Right Breathing in this category. There is one other big thing. We eat foods loaded with sugars and carbohydrates. Many people find relief by changing to a diet rich in dietary fats, proteins, and green leafy vegetables. Consider switching to a plant-based whole food diet or Dr. Perlmutter's modified ketogenic diet.

Techniques.

Let's call this DIY (do it yourself) Anxiety Management. Or DIYAM (pronounced Dam – the southern way). Many people see their doctor first. Maybe they try different medicines but don't get the relief and change they hope for. DIY.

How does it work? DIY is a bundle of technique options. All the options are good. The first step is a self-assessment. Am I anxious without a good cause? Do I want to live without anxiety? Do I want to get my life back under my control? Am I willing to do what it takes?[3]

If your answers are yes, yes, yes, and yes, then you are ready to take the next step.

Identify the problem. There is a little work involved. The books make it sound easy. "Explore and document the problem," they say. Fine. How?

Document as things happen. If you can, write things down. If tremors keep you from writing, use speech to text software to "write" things down. Writing things down helps. Pretend to be a reporter and gather the facts. Who, what, when, where, why, and how?

- Begin with what. What happened?
- When and where did it happen?
- Who else was involved?
- Why did it happen?
- How was it resolved?

Next, explore the problem. Did you resolve the issue to your satisfaction? If yes, what did you do that worked? Can you think of ways you could have fixed the problem better than you did? If so, write your preferred solution down. Can you think of other possible solutions? Jot them down too. Does one solution seem best for you? If so, plan to use it the next time this problem or a similar problem occurs.

Did that fix your anxiety problem? Probably not. You might need to do more. We recommend making The Golden Five the foundation for the way you live. Few people have heard of The Golden Five. But it is not a secret. The Golden Five have been hiding in plain sight our whole lives. Let us explain.

While researching movement disorders, including essential tremor (ET), the authors discovered time and again five unique elements. While recognized by others, the authors believe each item is useful if not critical for coping with ET and many additional problems.

The authors call these five essential elements The Golden Five. They are:

1)   Right Breathing

2)   Right Eating

3)   Right Exercising

4)   Right Sleeping

5)   Right Thinking

In the authors' opinions, The Golden Five form the foundation of every effort to achieve good health. Good health is the foundation for coping with movement disorders. Without good health, someone with essential tremor may have a difficult time marshaling the needed physical and mental resources.

The Golden Five is not just for this immediate audience. The women and men, mothers and fathers, even sisters and brothers who help can use The Golden Five to improve their health as well. When exercised and mastered The Golden Five can move anyone toward better overall health. Nothing is absolute, of course, so it is possible someone, somewhere, for some reason, might master all five elements or disciplines and yet still fail to improve his or her health. But that is not the way to bet.

A discipline is a field of study. In many disciplines, those who came before us uncovered truths had insights or created new knowledge we can use. Those willing to read widely may discover what we call The Golden Five. We uncovered the five disciplines quite by accident. While researching to write this book on movement disorders, we stumbled across bits and pieces of each discipline written in a few dozen books and perhaps a hundred papers. Nothing is original to the authors.

Let's begin with Right Breathing. The authors tried many different breathing techniques. Among the methods we tried was one we liked; intermittent breathing thoroughly explained in the book, *Breathe like a Master* mentioned earlier. Here are its essential steps.

Breathe only through the nose.

Breathe in naturally. Take slow, and soft breaths for some number of counts. Some books recommend a count of five. Steven discovered a four-count works best for him. Try different counts and keep what feels right for you.

Hold for some count. Steven holds for two counts. Others recommend a five-count.

Breathe out naturally. Breathe out slowly and softly. Steven breathes out for four counts.

Pause naturally. Steven pauses for one or two counts. Do what feels best for you. Different counts of in-hold-out-hold may come naturally at different times.

Next is Right Eating. Steven read four books and dozens of articles. For our purposes, consider eliminating all extra sugar from your diet. Cut way back on carbohydrates. Eat far more foods rich in dietary fats and proteins. Add mushrooms and leafy green vegetables to your meals. Cut back on how much you eat. Fast for a day once a week.

Right Exercising involves movement and activities. One should be up and moving around as much as possible. Try to walk a few hundred steps every hour. Get in at least 5,000 steps every day. Many people push for 10,000 daily steps. Steven discovered the simple addition of a smartwatch made it easy to walk, track, and increase his daily steps.

Right Sleeping is essential. It seems most of us need between seven and nine hours of sleep every day. Most westerners are sleep deficient. As Steven discovered, insufficient sleep leads to a wide variety of poor physical and mental health outcomes. Learn to get good sleep.

Right Thinking is the final discipline. At its simplest, our goal for Right Thinking is to deactivate our brain's default mode network (DMN) for a time each day. The DMN is where "we" go when we are not solving problems. Our mental states are more habitual than real. We guess about what is occurring. Our brains make up a great deal for efficiency's sake. We can disrupt the default mode through meditation and prayer. Both release serotonin, which makes us feel good.[4]

Chapter Twelve: Tinnitus

People who have essential tremor (ET) often discover they have tinnitus too. In an unscientific, informal survey on a Facebook essential tremor support group page, Greg's Story, tinnitus was the second most common additional complaint right after stress and anxiety.

Among the 25-30 million Americans who have tinnitus, a few things have emerged. The Mayo Clinic says tinnitus is more common among men than women, more common among smokers than non-smokers, and more common among people with diabetes than non-diabetics.

What is tinnitus? The Mayo Clinic calls tinnitus phantom noises. People with tinnitus hear a sound that does not exist outside the body.[1] The authors both have essential tremor and tinnitus. The sounds we hear do not exist outside of our heads.

We each experience tinnitus differently. For Steven, it is a soft, slowly rising rushing sound, almost electronic. Steven "hears" it in stereo, apparently originating behind his left ear. The sounds others hear include any simple sound. The American Tinnitus Association lists a variety of commonly reported sounds. Among them are clicks, ringing, buzzing, and hissing. And whistling, swooshing, and even roaring and screeching. Some people say they hear a pulsing or beating noise. Others describe chirping as the sound crickets make. Some people hear music.

Rose Peters, in her book, *Tinnitus the Thief of Silence*, reports that the sounds are not uniform. They vary in pitch and volume. They are more apparent when background sounds are low, for example, at night.[2] At night, tinnitus can be a real nuisance. Consider sleeping with quiet, soft, slow music playing. Steven tried a variety of music types before discovering that soft, slow, gentle, peaceful piano music works best for him. He also gains substantial relief from Tibetan Bowls.

The Center for Disease Control (CDC) claims about twenty-five million Americans have "experienced tinnitus… in the last year."[3] That is more than double the estimate for Americans with essential tremor. Not everyone who has essential tremor has tinnitus. And not everyone with tinnitus has essential tremor.

How do we "get" Tinnitus?

Many researchers believe it begins with hearing loss. The CDC reported during seven years from "2001-2008, an estimated 30 million Americans older than 12 years had hearing loss in both ears. An estimated 48 million had hearing loss in at least one ear."[4] As we live, we damage our ears. As we age, the damage accumulates. It is more common for people older than sixty. Sometimes we are exposed to loud noises. Some of us were near explosions or worked at airports. Sometimes we do it to ourselves. We may pump loud music into our ears through earbuds. Exposure to loud sounds over time can damage the tiny hairs in our inner ears. We can lose some of our hearing. High-frequency hearing loss is common.

Occasionally a buildup of ear wax might be the culprit. Sometimes our ear bones change.

What else can cause it? The American Academy of Otolaryngology provided a list beginning with noise-induced damage. Here are some other likely causes. It is a mouthful, but temporomandibular joint (TMJ) disorder may cause some cases of tinnitus. Head and neck injuries account for some examples. Middle ear infections and sinus infections can damage our hearing. Meniere's disease causes a buildup of fluids in the inner ear. With that comes a "stuffiness," dizziness, and other balance issues. Heart or blood vessel problems may result in a pulsing or beating noise. Some are common problems like atherosclerosis and high blood pressure. Others like turbulent blood flow and malformed capillaries are less common. Even certain medicines can damage the tiny hairs in our inner ears.[5]

As in every other area of life, some of the drugs and medicines we take may have side effects. If one takes twelve or more aspirin per day, tinnitus is more likely. Aspirin, ibuprofen, some cancer medicines, antidepressants, and even caffeine have been linked to tinnitus. So be careful out there.

Hearing loss and tinnitus are likely related.

We might be right to say it is all in our heads. We "hear" the sound in our ears. In the actual hearing, sound waves move tiny hairs inside our ears. Magically, our ear converts those movements into electrical signals. The auditory nerves move the signals into our brain, where the brain interprets the signals as sounds. The same nerves do other things as well. Tinnitus may involve our neural circuits misbehaving. Our brains are both complex and fragile.

In a study with a depressingly long name, Nathan Weisz, and four others argued that "the regional pattern of abnormal spontaneous activity we found could reflect a tinnitus-related cortical network."[6] What did they find? They found brain activity using magnetoencephalography, or MEG, in a group of individuals with tinnitus. The brain activity occurred "regionally." Regionally? More than one part of the brain lit up.

What do Nathan and his team believe occurs? In most cases, a person's auditory system is damaged. Think ear and associated nerves that carry the sound signals into the auditory portions of the brain. The sound "input" signals are changed, reduced, or even stopped. Uh-oh! Our brains don't like being shut out. So, our brains make things up. And we experience phantom sounds in our heads.

The good news is that we are not crazy. If we are insane, it is not due to tinnitus. People who experience tinnitus may also have sleep disorders, which bring more problems. We have fatigue, more stress, more anxiety, depression, and increased irritability. People may also have headaches and dizziness. Some even have memory loss.

Musical Ear Syndrome

Earlier, we mentioned that some people hear phantom music. It is common enough to have a name, musical ear syndrome (MES). The "go-to guy" for MES is Neil Bauman, Ph.D. Doctor Neil is an interesting guy in his own right. He has degrees in everything from forestry to astronomy to theology. Neil coined the term musical ear syndrome (MES) years ago in 2004. Since then, everyone, including this book's authors, reads what he has to say about MES specifically and tinnitus generally.

Musical ear syndrome (MES) is real. Well, not real, real. MES is Bauman's name for musical hallucinations. Researchers believe as many as 2% of people with hearing loss have MES. One friend who approached Steven said, "I was…glad it has a name, and maybe I am not crazy."

What music do people with MES "hear?" According to Doctor Neil, more than half hear Christmas carols and patriotic music. Remember, people with MES are hallucinating. Given that, why Christmas carols and patriotic music? Here is our guess. MES is more common in women than in men. The typical person with MES is 50 years old or older. It is more common in people older than 60. As a person older than 60, one of the authors remembers growing up with Christmas carols and patriotic music.[7] When today's younger people are older than 60, will they hallucinate Brittney Spears, Madonna, and rap music?

If you have MES, you have hearing loss. You are more likely to have this unusual version of tinnitus if you live alone in a quiet environment. If you are OCD (obsessive-compulsive disorder), you are more likely to hallucinate music. Here is more bad news. It is sometimes confused with dementia. In roughly two-thirds of the cases, MES is associated with drugs or alcohol, depression, dementia, and schizophrenia.

On one audiology website, some people with MES claimed they could change the music by thinking about it. One claimed to enjoy the music. Most said it disrupts conversations and makes it hard to enjoy a movie.

Carol Pestel wrote a paper, "Musical Ear Syndrome: What do we Know?" In it, she identifies some 368 drugs, herbs, and chemicals that can cause musical hallucinations. If you have

MES, it may be worth reading her paper to see if you are using any of the drugs or herbs she mentions.[8]

If you have MES, is there anything you can do about it? MES is a form of tinnitus. Doctor Neil recommends we all stop dwelling on our tinnitus. Some people claim it bothers them far less when they are busy working on something they want to do.

Can tinnitus be "fixed"? It doesn't seem like it. The way to bet is most solutions don't work. Tinnitus, after all, is a symptom.

One can find any number of dietary supplements recommended for treating tinnitus. There is no scientific evidence that any of them work. What can we do then? Rose Peters says, "Knowledge can change the life of a tinnitus sufferer."[9] How? We are not alone. We need not become isolated, lonely, and depressed. Others somehow cope. What else can we do?

We can pay better attention to the hearing we have left. Protect it. We can do things to mask tinnitus. During the day, we can use white noise generators. Use the key-phrase "in-ear white noise." One can find many options.

Additionally, one can buy a desktop white noise generator. One can use the desktop white noise generator at night, as well. Some people prefer forest sounds, thunderstorms, or rainstorms, while others prefer soft, slow, light piano, flute, or Tibetan bowl music.

One can find dozens of websites offering habituation methods claiming we can "get used to it" and therefore disregard it.

Chapter Thirteen: Sleep Disorders

In an informal Facebook survey, the author discovered that about one-third of all the people who have essential tremor recognize they don't sleep well. Many of us don't realize we have lived sleep-deprived most of our lives.

The authors first considered reading a few recommendations from medical advice websites like WebMD and Johns Hopkins, then compiling a shortlist of helpful tips on getting better sleep. After all, just how vital can sleep be to our problems?

We were wrong.

One thing led to another. One book led to another. And another. Ten books as of this writing. After the first few books, it became apparent that sleep is a big deal. So big a deal we added sleep to our Golden List, increasing it from Four to Five essential disciplines.

What do we know about sleep? We spend about one-third of our lives sleeping. Think about it. If we live to age 90, we can expect to sleep for a total of thirty years. Every day we spend about eight hours sleeping or trying to.

Why would we be designed to get so much sleep if sleep was not necessary? Sleep is vital. And most of us do not realize we don't get enough sleep. What is the right amount? Each of us is different. Children need more sleep because growth occurs during deep sleep. Adults require a little less. Our bodies spend deep sleep time repairing tissue damage, consolidating learning, and cleaning our brains. Seriously. A good range is from seven and a half hours to as many as nine hours. Most authors agree adults need 7.5 to 8 hours.

How do you know if you are not getting enough sleep? Sometimes, you just know. If you have trouble falling asleep or staying asleep, you are probably not getting enough sleep. If you have difficulty waking up in the morning or are a morning grouch, you are probably not getting enough sleep. If you feel lousy after you wake up, you are not getting enough sleep. Healthy sleep leaves us feeling good.

You may be thinking, "Never mind all that! Just tell me what to do!"

Okay. Several authors mentioned sleep hygiene. Sasha Stephens, in her book *The Effortless Sleep Method*, promises if you follow her rules, you will get more and better sleep (or as Sasha says, "you will recover").[1] We found her rules to be reasonable, if not unique.

Other authors delved into the science behind sleep and waking. Our favorite author is Dr. Kirk Parsley. His book, *Sleep to Win*, is both short and useful. Dr. Parsley recommends we learn to follow the sun. We used to fall asleep around three hours after sundown. He explains our retinal nerves are attuned to blue light. Light keeps us awake. When the sun sets, our nervous system, the nerve bundles in our eyes, sense the difference, and signals our brains that it is time to wind down and prepare to sleep.[2]

Here is what you need to know.

Build helpful sleep readiness habits. Our minds respond well to rituals. Wikipedia says, "A ritual is a sequence of activities involving gestures, words, and objects, performed in a sequestered place, and performed according to [a] set sequence."[3]

Each author we read approached what we choose to call sleep readiness in different ways. While individual parts are important, the ritual, the daily, disciplined, routine habit followed through consistently is as important. We think Dr. Parsley's discussion of blue light is the foundation of better sleep.

Here is our list of sleep readiness options for you to consider.

- Follow the sun. Reduce your exposure to blue light (almost all visible light) about three hours before you plan to sleep.
- Have a regular bedtime and stick to it.
- Try some light, slow stretching about an hour before bedtime.
- Meditate to slow your breathing.
- Turn off the TV news and talk radio about three hours before bedtime.
- Take a warm bath.
- Drink a cup of warm milk with a dab of honey.
- Cool the room temperature down.
- Listen to soft, restful music.
- Intend to get better, more restful sleep.
- Read yourself a bedtime story.
- Open a scent from a list people claim helps them to sleep. Chris Baird's list includes bergamot, chamomile, jasmine, lavender, and rose.[4]

Once you are ready to sleep, turn your room temperature down. Try different temperatures to find the one that is right for you. We have tried temperatures from 64 F to 67 F. Greg likes to sleep with his room temperature in the 50s! Steven sleeps best when the room temperature is 66 F. Be bold. If your feet get hot, stick them out from under the covers.

Turn off cell phones, tablets, laptops, and televisions. Keep your room dark and quiet. Turn on soft, light, easy listening music. Luis Bryan recommends calming, peaceful music, or nature sounds. Give quiet singing birds, gentle, flowing rivers, or swishing leaves a try.[5] Greg likes rain and thunderstorms. Steven has a sleep playlist consisting of soft, slow piano, quiet, slow flutes, and Tibetan bowls. Keep the volume low. Some people use a white noise generator.

For the longer term, invest in the right mattress and right pillow. Some suggest buying a new pillow every other year as they wear out as well as accumulating dust and other potential allergens.

If you drink alcohol, avoid drinking in the last three hours before sleeping. Steven loves his dark red wines and a small tray of cheeses. But cheese contains a stimulant, tyrosine, as does chocolate.[6] So Steven is gradually moving this guilty pleasure into the early evening.

Keep your bedroom clean and uncluttered.

There is quite a bit more one can do. If you are overweight, lose the extra weight. It can make a big difference. Re-examine the sections on stress and anxiety. Stress and anxiety have a significant impact on sleep. If you have pets, keep them off your bed. Cut down or eliminate late evening snacks—some, or perhaps many, of the foods we love cause alertness.

Be willing to use a trial and error method to find what works for you. For this to work, document what you are doing. Note any sleep improvements. Start with these ideas. If you like science, buy Dr. Parsley's book. It is a short, enjoyable read. If you just want a method without all the science, then buy Sasha Stephens' book.

Chapter Fourteen: Depression

In the informal Facebook group survey, some people with essential tremor complained they were depressed. Neither of your authors has experience with depression. But we love research. So, we spent two intense weeks researching depression and self-help techniques others claim have helped them. Here is what we found.

Depression is an inflammatory disorder that affects our moods.[1] One author described depression as a feeling of persistent sadness. The National Institute of Mental Health (NIMH) says it is a "common but serious mood disorder."[2] NIMH lists signs and symptoms they claim may indicate depression. The list is, well, depressing. Here are just a few of the symptoms they contain, persistent sad, anxious, or "empty" mood, feelings of hopelessness or pessimism, irritability, feelings of guilt, worthlessness, or helplessness. That is enough. If you think you may be depressed, find the link and look through the list.

None of the self-help books addressed what may be the most important single thing about depression. What we eat can change everything. The foods we eat and the drinks we drink alter the level of inflammation we experience in our bodies. A study published in May 2019 established a "clear causal link between dietary inflammation" and health problems, including diabetes, obesity, cardiometabolic disorders, and "increased risk of developing depression."[3] Increased inflammation is associated with "severe mental illnesses (SMI), including major depressive disorder, bipolar disorder, and schizophrenia."[4]

The connection between eating and health, including mental health, may change everything.

Is this medical science rock-solid? No. Not yet. However, Dr. Perlmutter claimed "higher levels of inflammation dramatically increase the risk of developing depression. And the higher the levels of inflammatory markers, the worse the depression."[5]

The Firth Review cited above showed the connection between what we eat and depression risks and severity. The reviewers created a dietary inflammation index to better link foods to inflammation levels. Not surprisingly, the study showed that diets high in saturated fats and carbs increase inflammation. Eating refined grains, processed meats, and drinking sugary soft drinks increases inflammation. High fiber diets packed with leafy greens and colorful vegetables lower inflammation.

What comes first? Poor diet or depression? For now, we can leave that interesting question to the doctors and scientists. It is clear a western diet loaded with saturated fats and carbs is associated with an increased risk of depression.[6] Other diet options, such as the plant-based Mediterranean diet of vegetables, nuts, beans, herbs, fruits, dairy, poultry, eggs and seafood, lower inflammation.[7] Dr. Perlmutter's modified ketogenic diet should also be considered.[8]

Inflammation is a problem. "Chronic and acute inflammation is thought to have a number of detrimental effects on brain structure and function, which, in turn, appear to adversely affect cognitive performance."[9] Too much sugar and too many carbohydrates may wreck your brain and turn you stupid. Or, as Dr. Perlmutter put it, "the higher the blood sugar, the faster the cognitive decline."[10] Altering your diet may be a smart move!

What else can we do to reduce inflammation and our risk of depression? The Firth Review discussed "the antidepressant effects of omega-3 fatty acids" and folate supplements.[11] We need at least 300 mg of Omega- 3 DHA every day to protect our brains. High levels of DHA correlated with lowered risks of Alzheimer's disease. If that wasn't enough reason to supplement with omega-3 DHA now, it is clear it also reduces our depression risks.

In addition to improving our diets by eliminating extra sugars and simple carbohydrates, we should also consider getting a bit more exercise.

The beta-blocker, Propranolol, occasionally increases one's chance of becoming depressed or worsening depression. Keep in mind that most people are treated for more than one condition. The interactions of your medications could increase your chances of becoming depressed. This includes both prescribed and over-the-counter medicines and herbs.

While researching the role of side-effects, the authors discovered the epigenetic role of childhood stress on lifelong risks of depression. Children who experienced high-stress levels early in life may be predisposed to depression (and suicide) for the rest of their lives. This may worsen medicines' side effects concerning depression. Discuss your stress history with your doctor.

Consider a layered approach. Always talk to your doctor as an essential first step. Your doctor can help you assess your depression. Use medicines for immediate relief. Change your diet from the Western diet that is killing you to a plant-based diet. Use a few dietary supplements. Add in some daily exercise. Then add in some of the hundreds of self-help techniques that are available. There are hundreds of inexpensive self-help books from which to choose.

Here is a short list of treatment options and self-help tips from a sampling of books we found. Remember, always talk to your doctor:

- Acceptance and Commitment Therapy (ACT)
- Cognitive Behavioral Therapy (CBT) CBT intends to help one gain perspective about the past and the future. Add CBT to other treatments to improve treatment outcomes.[12]
- Mindfulness-Based Stress Reduction (MBSR)
- Meditation and Prayer. A new area called neurotheology shows spiritual experiences change one's mind. "People who spend hours in prayer and meditation are actually different."[13]
- Exercise. A Harvard study showed sustained, low-intensity exercise is beneficial in reducing depressive symptoms. Exercise supports nerve cell growth in the hippocampus.[14]
- Aromatherapy
- Develop good daily habits.
- Keep a journal.
- Take a walk in the sunshine and a nature setting.
- Stay off social media like Facebook, Twitter, and Instagram.
- And hundreds more.

Chapter Fifteen: Dizziness

From time to time, each of us experiences something we call dizziness. We use the word dizziness to describe a range of sensations. When we sit up in bed quickly or stand up immediately, we may momentarily feel lightheaded. We may feel faint, become unsteady, or lose our balance. We may say we feel woozy.

Some of us describe it as a feeling of turning in space. Alternatively, we are still while all of the space spins rapidly around us. Others describe dizziness as a floating or swimming sensation.

Many people who have essential tremor also complain of dizziness.[1] It is not just people with ET. Around one-fifth of us get dizzy in any given year.[2] Dizziness is far more common than ET.

Why do we, people who have essential tremor, get dizzy? People who see their doctors for ET tend to be older. People who see their doctors because they are dizzy also tend to be older. Both populations tend to use multiple medications routinely. In many cases, the medicines we use to treat other symptoms may have a slight amount of dizziness as a side effect. For example, Propranolol, commonly used to treat ET lists "dizziness, faintness, or lightheadedness when getting up suddenly from a lying or sitting position" as a side effect.[3] Primidone, another drug commonly prescribed for people with ET, lists "dizziness or lightheadedness," "sensation of spinning," clumsiness or unsteadiness," and a "feeling of constant movement of self or surroundings."[4] Now add both together.

We get dizzy because we are humans subject to all the usual human conditions. And dizziness is a symptom of many other diseases, disorders, injuries, and infections. If something affects one's ears, brain, or blood flow, expect to be dizzy from time to time.

Given all that, what can we do? Make a list of every medicine and supplement you take. Using your favorite search engine search for the side effects of each drug. Note the ones that list any of the dizziness symptoms. If you drink alcohol, be sure to add it to your list. Then talk to your doctor. Your doctor may change your prescriptions if you are stacking dizziness side effects.

Surprise! Right eating and right exercising can both help. Our brains and blood flow change based on our diets and how much exercise we get. Moving away from our western diet toward a plant-based diet can improve one's blood flow and protect one's brain. Limiting salt and caffeine may also lessen dizziness episodes.

Dear Reader, did you know you have rocks in your head? Our ears rely on tiny calcium carbonate crystals to help us figure out gravity. Sometimes the crystals, or rocks, break free and move from where they are supposed to be to a place where they are not welcome. When they break free and move, they can cause us to feel as if we are spinning. We call it vertigo.

For recurring vertigo, ask your doctor about the Epley Maneuver.[5] No, it isn't something one would find in an old Star Trek episode. It is a way of moving your head. It can help to move those "rocks" to a more suitable place in your ear. The best part is that it can be done at home.

Chapter Sixteen: Stammering, Embarrassment, and Isolation

Stammering or stuttering.

Stammering or stuttering is another common complaint among those of us who have essential tremor. Let's begin with what stammering is. Researchers call it a speech disorder. One can find stutterers among people of all ages. A description we found useful says it is speech with involuntary breaks or halts and frequently includes "spasmodic repetitions of sounds or syllables."[1]

Stuttering has its own jargon. Developmental stuttering (DS) is the most common form. For the most part, DS involves children who stutter (CWS). Note the number of acronyms. As many as 10% of children stutter. DS begins as early as 18 months of age, with almost all onsets between children, ages two to four. This age range parallels when speech development occurs.[2] Nearly all children who stutter stop stuttering during childhood. Far more females naturally recover than do males.[3]

In general, stuttering begins far earlier than essential tremor.

Stuttering affects less than 1% of the population. Researchers estimate ET affects about 4% of us. Given those numbers, one should rarely find someone who stutters who also has essential tremor. Why does it seem that so many people with ET stutter? Maybe the two disorders are related. In an informal survey, people with ET said they stuttered almost as often as they complained of dizziness and sleep disorders.[4]

Persistent developmental stuttering begins in childhood. It continues into adulthood.

Why do we stutter? We don't know. Persistent developmental stuttering in adulthood or adults who stutter (AWS) is strongly associated with anxiety. Essential tremors is also strongly associated with anxiety. Dr. Perez offers several clues in his paper. He cites differences between people who stutter and those who do not "specifically in the auditory and motor regions and the basal ganglia" in our brains. Also, there is "abnormal coordination between brain areas that plan and coordinate speech."[5]

Is there a "cure" for stuttering? If there is, we did not find one mentioned. Many approaches have been tried with varying degrees of success. What has been tried? Medicines. Anti-psychotics take about eight weeks to show effect. The studies are small. Then we have both alcohol and cannabis. The evidence is anecdotal. Reddit has a /Stutters subreddit (a group) where a few people discussed how a small amount of alcohol or marijuana reduced their stuttering. The same people said more than a little worsens stuttering.[6]

Other approaches include alternative medicines like acupuncture. It is unclear that any of the natural remedies work. They seem to focus on anxiety reduction strategies. If trying these strategies appeals to you, take another look at Chapter Six on anxiety and Chapter Nine on depression.

J. Scott Yaruss makes several additional suggestions, including using electronic devices to help slow speech, thus enhancing fluency as well as self-help and support groups. According to Yaruss, "self help and support groups…play a prominent role for recovery for many people who stutter."[7]

Embarrassment and Isolation.

We visibly tremble. We drop things. We spill food and drinks. We are embarrassed because we are not "normal." We have other problems in addition to essential tremor that make our situation even worse. We are anxious, stressed, and maybe depressed. We are uncomfortable in public. People stare. We stop going out. We stay at home. We isolate ourselves.

Isolation can lead to loneliness. Loneliness, in turn, can become deep sadness.

How do we turn things around?

We must first decide what we want. We gradually stopped doing things. Slowly begin doing things again. Find a support group. Do things together.

Chapter Seventeen: Things we wish

These are some of the things we wish a gifted designer, inventor, or engineer would develop.

Blue jeans and slacks with large pockets. When we tremble, we may want big pockets to put our hands in. Add separate pockets for our cell phones and keys.

Game programmers write your game interfaces to include options for people with movement disorders to play. We have trouble with mouse movements and keyboard controls.

Create eating utensils to help us move food from a plate or bowl to our mouths without spilling all over ourselves. This is a big deal. Don't build us something that looks peculiar.

Design kitchen cutting systems to help us prepare foods without cutting our fingers.

Build a coffee cup that will not slosh nor spill. Try not to make it look like something a two-year-old would drink from.

Build tablet and cell phone cases we can hold without dropping.

Build writing pens to restore our once excellent handwriting.

Design key and lock systems people with movement disorders can use.

Design cell phone and tablet interfaces that understand our trembling might not mean we intended to type five "a"s in a row. Consider that people who have movement disorders need to input phone numbers. Make it easy.

Design speech to text software to seamlessly interact with social media web sites like Facebook.

Design computer keyboards with movement disorder options. Let us tune it to our needs. Some people need just a little extra help. Others are unable to use keyboards today.

Design computer mice that learn what we intend to do.

Design or invent brilliant zippers, buttons, snaps, and shoelaces.

Design a brilliant razor able to compensate for our trembling.

Many of us need help pouring liquids like milk. We want something better than a large funnel.

Design small tools able to compensate for trembling.

Design food cans/containers people with movement disorders can easily open.

Design smart, wearable wrist weights. Make it possible to adjust the amount of weight quickly and easily.

Design everything else with movement disorders in mind.

Conclusion

Essential tremor lasts a lifetime. Spend time understanding it. Try different techniques to help you cope with the new challenges you face. Join support groups and pass on what works for you.

As we finished up this book, we thought about our situations. We are brothers but we grew up in different worlds. We asked ourselves what advice we would give to our younger selves, the men we were before essential tremor, to help prepare our older selves to cope better with our movement disorder. Here is what we came up with:

Develop a good character.

Don't complain. Complaining does not add, it subtracts. But do ask for alternatives.

Be grateful. First, enjoy your life. It is yours. Many of us have no idea how to do this. We suggest beginning with an inventory. We call them personality statements, or "I am" statements. No one needs to see your statements. Steven begins his personality statements with, "People say that I am." Here are a few starters. People say that I am loyal, kind, considerate, smart… you get the idea. Go wild. Next, write down "I like" statements. People say that I like…here are some starters. People say that I like chocolates, strange coffee concoctions, reading, learning, writing, emotional music, musicals, cats, raccoons and skunks, World of Warcraft (it is a computer game), and junk (if I didn't like junk I would keep less of it around). Enjoy the big things and the little things. Say thank you. Say thank you a lot. No, really. Say thank you.

Be nice. Be gentle with yourself. Be gentle with and think about others. Unless you are a judge, don't judge others. We all make our choices for our own reasons. Don't blame people for making different choices. Be as helpful as you can. Try (really try) not to insult people.

Accept that life will not be fair. While you will struggle, it can be useful for you. We struggle best when we have a wide choice of tools to choose from. Movement disorders find a way to disrupt some things we enjoy doing. It can stop some things, but not everything. First on our list is learn! If you can, learn something new every day. Notice, this isn't every day for a week, or a month or even a year. Learn something new about things, about people, and about yourself every day for the rest of your life. Learn from your mistakes and from the mistakes others make. Learn skills. Can you make things? Great! Can you teach things? Excellent. Take more risks. Discover what it is you want and act. Learn to lead. Begin by setting a good example. Insofar as possible, learn to be self-reliant.

In this short list, we will end with this. Spend as much time as you can with people you enjoy and love. For most people, this means spending more time with your family. If you don't have a family or don't like your family, meet new people, get to know them and make your own family. Spend less time around negative people. Turn off the television news. And limit your daily exposure to talk radio.

Oh, one more thing. A few years ago, when we were growing up, in 1967, some great philosophers sang some good advice. At least consider what The Grass Roots said.

Let's Live for Today

When I think of all the worries

People seem to find.

And how they're in a hurry

To complicate their minds.

By chasing after money

And dreams that can't come true.

I'm glad that we are different,

We've better things to do.

May others plan their future,

I'm busy loving you.

1-2-3-4

Sha-la-la-la-la-la,

live for today.

Sha-la-la-la-la-la,

live for today.

And don't worry 'bout tomorrow,

Hey, hey, hey.

Sha-la-la-la-la-la,

live for today.

Live for today.

Before you go…we rely on your reviews to drive interest and sales. If you loved this book, *The Hand I was Dealt*, please go to Amazon and write a short review. Give us plenty of stars. And tell everybody.

If you hated it just tell your mother-in-law.

For those of you interested in Steven's first book the first two chapters are included here:

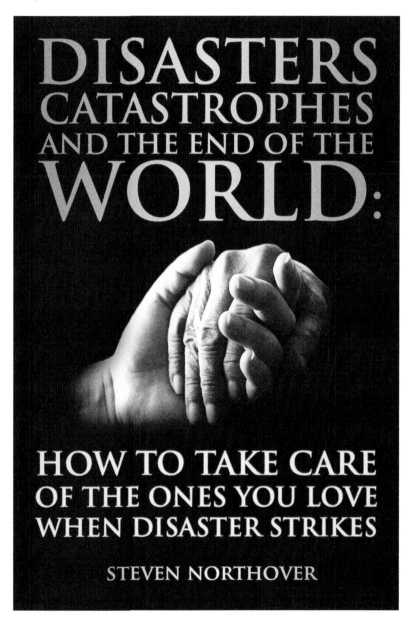

Introduction

Every week a disaster or catastrophe happens somewhere. Every week, people like you and me are caught unready to meet these life-endangering challenges. You might think you don't have the time, energy, effort, and money to get and stay ready. But what if I told you that you can have what Preppers have, the supplies and the skills, without doing much more than you are already doing? After all, that is what you want, isn't it? You want to be your family's First Responder when no one else is coming. This book, *Disasters, Catastrophes, and the End of the World* will help you get and stay ready in less time, using less energy and less money than if you do it on your own. I wrote this book to help you rapidly evolve, step by step, from someone who is not prepared for disasters to someone confident in their abilities to handle whatever comes. Read and follow these simple steps. You will know what to plan for, what to do, and how to prepare to survive the disasters you are likely to face.

Who am I to help you get ready? I am someone much like you. I lived through a disaster a few years ago. I was an engineering manager with one of the major defense corporations. I saw how unprepared most people were. I saw how people muddled through without water, food, and power. Before that, I served as an Army officer for twenty years. Now, I spend my time learning about human problems and how to solve them. Because I have spent my time thinking, studying, and planning, I am the perfect person to guide you. I can save you time. I can save you effort. And I can show you what you can accomplish on your tight budget. You will be surprised at how a little additional effort applied every week for a few weeks can increase your confidence in your ability to lead your family at a time when it counts the most.

If you are like most people today, you are busy juggling everything you must already do. You probably have a job where you work too hard for too little money. When you are not at work you must shop, clean, take care of children and pets. You barely have time to socialize. How will you fit in one more thing? I understand. I will make it as easy as I can for you to be ready without becoming a prepper.

In a couple of pages, in Chapter One, I will discuss disasters from our past. You will gain a sense of what has happened, and therefore, what could happen. I will describe planning in Chapter Two, what it is, why it is helpful, and what to plan for based on where you live today. You will learn about what the government intends to do and what it says you must do for yourself.

Then, I will discuss things you will want to think about as you prepare. I will guide you, in Chapter Three, to help you think about planning for your health and physical fitness, as well as your emotional and economic fitness. I will help you to develop your plan to lead your family when no help comes. And if no one is coming for a while, I will help you think about how to care for yourself and your family until help does eventually arrive.

After surviving through the damage phase of a disaster, you may need first-aid supplies. In Chapter Four, I will help you plan for first aid. I will show you some options that worked for me to build a shelter-in-place first-aid kit. In addition to these supplies, you will need water and food. In Chapter

Five, I will help you to plan ahead so you will have enough of each. When you plan ahead, you will see that some skills you don't have today could be quite helpful to have in a disaster situation. In Chapter Six, I will offer suggestions for how to get those skills or how to join with others who have them.

At this point, you may be wondering what is in Chapter Seven. There, I will help you to build and maintain your family's Disaster Survival Plan.

Just for fun, in Chapter Eight, I will take you through possible, and unlikely, world endings. Well, it would be "The End of the World as We Know It." No, not the song, the way we experience our world today. If you are ready for the Zombie Apocalypse, you will be fine for lesser scenarios.

In Chapter Nine, I will briefly discuss recovery for when the disaster has ended, and it is time to return to a normal life once again. In Chapter Ten, I offer some final words.

Who is this book for?

If you want to be prepared without becoming a prepper, this book is for you. If you don't have the time or simply do not wish to read dozens of books and search hundreds of web sites for the basics, this book is for you. If you want a good reason (or two or three or five) to plan, this book is for you. If you want someone to guide you through the first necessary steps to preparedness, this book is for you. This book is for the busy person who wants a guide to show them what to do and why to do it, with the smallest amount of time, energy, effort, and money. This book will be for those who want to prepare for the most likely disasters, those where the utility companies restore power in a month or less.

This book is for the person who knows that sometimes we are called upon to be the hero.

Who is this book not for?

This book is not for preppers. If you are a prepper, you have already prepared and documented your plan. You already know your health as well as the health of those you have taken responsibility for. You are physically fit or well on your way. You have already thought about the difficult questions and have your own answers to them. Economically, you are well on your way to freedom. You have enough cash on hand to make it through thirty days without help. You have individual first-aid kits and a Disaster First-Aid Kit tailored to the number of people you plan to take care of. You have all the skills you need to survive, and even thrive, when no help comes in that first month. You are self-reliant in most aspects of your life. For you, being a prepper is a lifestyle choice.

Purpose of the book

I wrote this book to help you think through the three key days of a disaster. The day before, when you have all the time you need to think and prepare. The day of, when your goal is to survive with no injuries or illnesses. And the day after, when you must care for those who need you and attempt to return to the new normal.

If you follow this guide, you will be far better prepared to handle any short-term disaster or long-lasting catastrophe than you are today. If you are a husband, a wife, a parent, someone who cares for another person, or a leader in your daily life, use this guide, follow it to help you be a rock in a time of trouble. Choose to be ready. You can make a difference.

Don't miss out on the opportunity to prepare ahead of time for disasters yet to come. Don't be one of those people who suddenly finds themselves in the midst of a catastrophe they are unprepared to handle. Instead, buy this inexpensive guide, read it, and begin your preparations. There will always be another catastrophe. You owe it to yourself, and those who rely on you, to be ready.

Ch. 1 A Brief History of Disasters

In this chapter, I will cover the most serious disasters that you could be exposed to. I will give real-life examples and help you make decisions about what to prepare for. I have lived through two disasters, a flood and a flurry of tornadoes. Like most people, I was not ready. Learn from my study and experiences. Then, what happened to me will not happen to you and your family.

We do not prepare for disasters. Most of us live day-to-day with little thought for how we will cope when the inevitable disaster occurs. Fortunately, most disasters are short-lived. Local governments arrive with water, first aid, and police support. Sometimes, they come with cash cards. Help almost always comes in the first couple of days, but not always.

Life exposes usto a variety of disasters and catastrophes. Where we live changes the kinds of disasters we are most likely to experience. There are no safe places. I looked at a wide variety of sources, using the Internet to create a disaster list. I read dozens of pages and could have read hundreds more to develop this list with examples. This list begins with the most deadly disaster, floods, followed by hurricanes and tornadoes. After floods, hurricanes, and tornadoes, the list is in alphabetical order.

Floods

I was surprised to discover that floods are big events. I suppose I should have known it. Noah, if we believe the account in the Old Testament, experienced an extraordinary disaster. For everyone involved, it was the end of the world as they knew it. In a later chapter, I will discuss those kinds of world-ending disasters.

In the United States, floods cause more losses than any other type of disaster. Floods account for less than half of all disasters, yet they do nearly all the damage.[1] Last year, South Carolina was underwater. Their flood came from rains. CNBC reported more than a million gallons of water per person, with a total of more than eleven trillion gallons of rain, fell on North and South Carolina.[2] As I write this chapter, flood waters cover large parts of Louisiana and Mississippi.

China has been devastated by floods, both historically and recently. In 1887, the Yellow River flooded. Fifty thousand square miles were affected. Between one and two million people died from the flood or its aftermath. The Yangtze River flood, in 1931, claimed between one and four million lives from drowning, disease, and starvation. In 1975, the Banqiao Dam collapsed. Twenty-six thousand were killed that day. Up to one hundred thousand more died from disease and famine.

You must survive the flood and then deal with contaminated water and the lack of food.

Hurricanes

In the United States, hurricanes are the second most damaging kind of disaster. Here are four examples: In

[1] P. 530 Koenig and Schultz's Disaster Medicine: Comprehensive Principles and Practices.
[2] http://www.cnbc.com/2015/10/08/south-carolinas-rain-and-floods-by-the-numbers.html

Galveston, Texas, in 1900, the tidal surge caused by a hurricane killed at least six thousand people. Hurricane Andrew, in 1992, killed sixty-five people in Florida and caused twenty-six billion dollars in damages. Hurricane Katrina, in 2005, damaged large swaths of the Gulf Coast, including New Orleans. Many local governments, including the state government of Louisiana, were overwhelmed and failed. The US federal government found its own response inadequate. Eighty billion dollars in losses occurred.

Tornadoes

In 2011, hundreds of tornadoes blew their way across twenty states in the US in a few days. Where I live in Alabama experienced significant damage and a loss of electrical power for about five days.

High winds and water caused many immediate injuries and long-term problems. Bodily high-wind injuries included blunt force trauma, which caused deep bruises, broken bones, dislocated shoulders, punctured lungs, and many lacerations. Water further damaged structures and contaminated some of the water supplies.

Disease

I don't know why, but I am not concerned about this one. The 1918 Spanish Flu epidemic did kill enormous numbers of people. The lower death estimate I found was twenty million people. Stay as healthy as you can. Keep your shots up to date.

Earthquakes

Before my research, I believed earthquakes did the most damage, killed the largest numbers of people, and resulted in the greatest losses. Earthquakes get lots of press time. The pictures of the destruction grip our attention. The list of the recent biggest ones is impressive. The San Francisco earthquake in 1906 killed three thousand people and started fires that burned more than four square miles of the city. Chinese cities were hit several times by powerful earthquakes, once in 1920 and again in 1976. Between the two earthquakes, about half a million souls perished. An earthquake knocked down large portions of an interstate highway in Northridge, California, in 1994. California is an expensive place to have an earthquake. Authorities claimed twenty-five billion dollars in losses. Other earthquakes, in the Indian Ocean, Pakistan, Haiti, New Zealand, and Japan, all did enormous damage, with many dead and injured. The last one, in Japan, was 9.0 on the Richter scale. The resulting tsunami killed or injured about fifteen million people. A quarter of a million buildings were damaged or destroyed.

Earthquakes result in many crushing wounds, blunt force traumas, broken bones, and even burns. If water is involved, add compromised water supplies.

Heat waves

Heat waves occur more frequently than I realized. Two heat waves occurred recently in the US, one in 1980 and a second in 2010. At least five thousand people died. There were three European heat waves, in 2003, 2006, and 2010. All told, 125,000 people died. A heat wave becomes dangerous when combined with another disaster that cuts off electrical power.

Ice storms

We, in the United States, experience localized ice storms regularly. An ice storm coupled with high winds or coming at an unexpected time can be deadly. The ice storms I found listed all had light casualties, but sometimes the effects were surprising. In one case, a sudden temperature drop combined with high winds up to eighty miles per hour killed 140 people. Extreme cold weather coupled with a loss of electrical power could devastate a county, state or region.

Terrorism and industrial accidents

Terrorist attacks tend to affect only a local area and a few people. Terrorists adjust tactics as we thwart them. At this moment, attacks seem to be performed by individuals or small teams. Many involve homicide vests, small arms fire, and knives. We have seen attacks against train stations where multiple bombs or a dispersed chemical nerve agent killed dozens and injured thousands.

Industrial accidents tend to be localized events. Most involve explosions, gasses, fumes, or corrosive materials. Most affect only a small number of people.

Other disasters

There are other disasters we should consider. In the last several years, we have seen grass fires, forest fires, mudslides, and avalanches. The fires can move quickly and do substantial damage over large areas.

Now take a moment to think about four more disasters. The four disasters listed below are not listed above, because they make us uncomfortable. One is a recurring, natural event.

The other three are the result of enemy actions. These are Black Swan events. They are as unlikely in real life as your chance of seeing a black swan. Or are they? I offer them for your consideration.

Coronal Mass Ejection (CME)

CME is fascinating. The Sun routinely ejects enormous amounts of matter. The fastest CME can travel the distance from the Sun to the Earth in half a day. Most CMEs travel much slower, and nearly every single one misses the Earth. If one hits the Earth, it causes the Earth's magnetic field to slosh back and forth, creating massive current flows. Over the last several years, more authors believe a CME could devastate the North American electrical grid. Damage to the power grid and electrical systems is expected to be greatest in northern latitudes. Following a CME direct hit, we could be without electrical power for many months, possibly even for years.

Electromagnetic pulse (EMP)

An electromagnetic pulse (EMP) occurs when a nuclear weapon detonates. A nuclear weapon detonated at high altitude will result in little to no damage from thermal radiation or blast. The damage we experience will come from its EMP. Like the CME, it causes current to flow in electrical devices. This current flow can burn the wires, breaking them, thus destroying the devices. Who would use nuclear weapons in this way against us? North Korea, Iran, China, and Russia could. If a ballistic missile arrived over the center of the USA from our southern border, we might not see it coming. Iran has ballistic missiles. They have the desire. Do they have the EMP warhead they need? I believe they do or soon will have one. As with the CME, we could be without electrical power for many months. Many electrical devices would have to be replaced.

Cyber-physical attack

I believe this is the most likely attack. There are about one hundred electrical substations that convert power moved across long distances to power suitable for local distribution. Of those one hundred substations, thirty have been identified as crucial to the system. A few years ago, after the attack at the Metcalf Substation outside San Jose, California, *The Wall Street Journal* reported that the destruction of as few as nine substations out of the thirty would collapse the electrical grid.[3] The Metcalf Substation was the right kind of substation for this attack. A small number of attackers used aimed rifle fire to damage the massive transformers. It is more than a year later, and the FBI has no arrests and no suspects. On the cyber side, electrical power equipment is managed or monitored by devices called industrial control systems. A cyber-attack could cause these devices to malfunction in ways that have destroyed a generator in a test. There are many stories of nation-states like China and Russia penetrating the network facing side of our critical infrastructure, including the electrical grid. I believe this kind of cyber-attack is more likely now than ever before.

A successful cyber-physical attack, combining widespread cyber-attacks with physical attacks on specific locations, could destroy enough of the large transformers and other

---

[3]http://www.wsj.com/articles/SB10001424052702304020104579433670284061220

equipment to make it a multi-year effort to restore some electrical power to some users.

All three of these cases, the CME, EMP, or a cyber-physical attack, could collapse the electrical grid in ways that would make it difficult to restore. After the grid collapses, there will be no clean water, no sewage systems, no financial services, no transportation, no fuels, no communications, no food, no manufacture and distribution, and no news or entertainment. If this list is missing anything, there won't be any of whatever I missed either. The single biggest difference between the three is that the cyber-physical attack will not harm personal electronics nor vehicles.

Let's assume the worst. Let's assume a hostile nation, like Iran or North Korea, launches a ballistic missile that flies over the South Pole, approaching the US from the south. The enhanced electromagnetic pulse (EMP) warhead detonates a few hundred miles above the center of the North American continent. An EMP traveling at the speed of light would blanket the US and Canada from horizon to horizon. In the time it takes to draw in a deep breath, nearly everything with embedded chips would burn out. Enormous current flows will break long-haul electric lines. This attack may come with no warning.

Reasonable people have estimated that up to 90% of Americans would die in the first year without power. Many would become sick from waterborne diseases or die from starvation, medical problems, or criminal violence. My intuition tells me that the survivors will be the ones who prepare, plan, and organize with their neighbors.

In summary, we discussed the most dangerous disasters we face based on history. We also considered disasters that are frequently in the news, like wildfires, and finally, human-caused combat actions that could significantly impact us.

In the next chapter, I will make the case for planning and preparing to be self-sufficient, at first for three days, then for a week, and finally for a month.

Ch. 2 What is planning and why do I need to plan?

Dwight D. Eisenhower, the WWII Supreme Allied Commander for the invasion of Europe, stated, "In preparing for battle I have always found that plans are useless, but planning is indispensable." He also said, "Plans are nothing; planning is everything."

In the previous chapter, I discussed the most likely disasters. In this chapter, I want to show you the value planning has to offer in helping you prepare to cope and survive a disaster. I will introduce you to themes that I will flesh out throughout the rest of this book.

If you are a husband, wife, father, mother, or someone who cares for another person, then you will want to plan to deal with crises. Nearly all of us will experience disasters at some point in our lifetimes. With a good guide, we can prepare for most of them with a little effort and a little money. This chapter is a guide to most of the rest of the book. Subsequent chapters will cover each of my recommendations in more detail. If you follow this plan, you will be far better prepared to deal with the most likely disasters you may experience. You will be ready, and you will be more confident.

Most of us don't know what to do to prepare. Maybe you have considered buying one of those expensive emergency food plans. Think of it, you can store plastic buckets full of food in your basement for the next twenty-five years. But you won't be any better off than you are today. If you fail to plan, you missed the point.

Preparation begins with planning. The purpose of planning is to deliberately and methodically think through and document what you will do, what you will need, and what decisions you will have to make before, during, and immediately following a disaster or long-lasting catastrophe. It is more than just buying some plastic buckets full of food.

What should we plan for? We should prepare for the most common occurrences in the places we live. If you have lived in the same location for a while, you already know what kinds of disasters are most likely to happen. When I moved to Alabama, I asked people who lived here. Those who lived here all their lives told me tornados and lightning storms were a big problem. A few old-timers said it is those two days in the winter when snow falls and ice forms on the roads, and a mild insanity sets in. My planning accounts for lightning, tornados, and the mild insanity. Your planning should account for the disasters that are common where you live.

Most disasters are weather-related, caused by human error and accidents, or due to enemy actions. Weather includes extremes of heat and cold, high winds, rains and droughts, tornados and hurricanes, electrical storms, and ice storms. Space weather, a new field, includes solar flares and coronal mass ejections. And then there are the earthquakes, tsunami, and volcanic eruptions. Human error and accidents are unpredictable, other than to say that when they occur, they make some other problem worse and at the worst possible time. Enemy actions include terrorism, conventional acts of war, cyber-attacks, and nuclear attacks including electromagnetic pulse weapons.

As we prepare for disasters, how much preparation is reasonable? Most disasters will last for a day, a week, or maybe a few weeks. Some may last longer than a few weeks. For me, today, I plan to be self-sufficient for a month. That includes first aid, body temperature management, water, food, individual-specific needs such as medicines, and physical security. It includes physical, emotional, and economic fitness. It includes a primary plan to shelter in place, as well as alternate plans for fleeing the area by vehicle or walking out if necessary. You may not want to be a prepper, but you do want to be ready.

This chapter will provide an overview of the things we should think about as we plan. Some things are obvious. Everyone needs to consider the basics first. We all need adequate insurance. Insurance transfers some of our risks to others for a fee. Most of us have auto insurance, and homeowners have home insurance. Make sure they are adequate. Many homeowner's insurance policies do not cover floods. I mentioned that floods cause the most losses. In 2015, South Carolina had a flood when eleven trillion gallons of rain fell on it and North Carolina. In addition to auto and home insurance, most of us who are responsible for others need life insurance and disability insurance. Strange things happen. I didn't feel well one day, so I left work and went home. I crawled into bed. My wife convinced me I should go to the emergency room to be checked. I went and the next thing I knew, I could not return to work without a cardiologist's approval. Fortunately, I had both short-term and long-term disability insurance. I was not able to go back to work for two weeks. I was fine.

Being in the best possible health is extraordinarily important all the time, but especially during a disaster. The longer the self-help phase of a disaster lasts, the more important good health is. So be an adult. Schedule regular checkups and know the state of your health. I not only give advice, I take it. I recently had a complete battery of clinical tests. The tests showed me I am overweight (technically obese) and my cholesterol lingers at the high end of normal. My disaster planning addresses both issues.

As you plan, keep in mind how the people covered by your planning affect your options. For each one, think about their age, fitness, and health. Think about each person's capabilities and limitations. If someone in your group has special needs, think about what you will do to ensure they will manage. Each person's needs will be different. Be sure to think through what you will need and make arrangements now.

You should plan for fitness. Physical fitness is essential. Most of us are unfit and unready to deal with the stresses that come from the long-lasting catastrophes. All too often we sit, eat, and drink too much when we should be up and moving. If you are like me, you might have to learn how to walk correctly. You will need to learn and train to carry what you need. Your physical tasks during a crisis may increase. Begin preparing now.

Fitness includes emotional fitness. Know yourself. Do you have the ability to see and understand what is occurring around you? Do you recognize danger as it builds? Do you have a survivor's mind? How well do you handle stress? Have you thought through what you will do in a disaster when people come looking for food, first aid, and shelter?

What will you do if you or your family members are threatened? Will you defend yourself? Can you use deadly force? Or will you run? Thinking through these questions now will help you make better decisions when things are uncertain, and time is short.

Fitness also includes economic fitness. If a disaster or a prolonged catastrophe happens, your access to your money and credit may be limited. The place you work may be closed. If power is out, you might not be able to use debit or credit cards. Cash or barter may be your only options.

Interested? To buy this book Search Amazon for:

Disasters, Catastrophes, and the End of the World

Chapter Notes

Chapter One

[1] This story was first published at alwaysheadingnorth.com with the title Thank God, It's Friday!

Chapter Two

[1] This story was first published at alwaysheadingnorth.com with the title Filing For Unemployment.

Chapter Three

[1] This story was first published at alwaysheadingnorth.com with the title Essential Tremors at the July 4th Celebration.

Chapter Four

[1] This story was first published at alwaysheadingnorth.com with the title Fishing Before Essential Tremors.

[2] This story was first published at alwaysheadingnorth.com with the title Way of The River – Greg's Story.

[3] This story was first published at alwaysheadingnorth.com with the title Essential Tremors, The River, and the Fisherman.

Chapter Five

[1] This story was first published at alwaysheadingnorth.com with the title Before Essential Tremors – A Bear Surprise!

[2] This story was first published at alwaysheadingnorth.com with the title Before Essential Tremors – Fishing – Called to The River.

Chapter Six

[1] This story was first published at alwaysheadingnorth.com with the title

---

Essential Tremors, The Fisherman, and The River.

Chapter Seven

[1] Recollections based on conversations between March 2019 and November 2019 (Greg and Steven Northover).

Chapter Eight

[1] www.essentialtremor.org/about-et/ ET is often confused with Parkinson's disease, although it's eight times more common, affecting an estimated 10 million Americans and millions more worldwide.

Chapter Nine

[1] Medline Plus.gov

[2] Conversations via Facebook Messenger between the individuals and the author, Steven Northover during 2018 and 2019. See the Facebook group Essential Tremors - Self Help and Support - Greg's Story.

[3] Adapted from a story first published at alwaysheadingnorth.com with the title Movement Disorder Doctor Visit Guide – Intro.

[4] www.essentialtremor.org/about-et/ Essential tremor (ET) is a neurological condition that most commonly causes a rhythmic trembling of the hands while performing a task such as eating, writing, dressing, drinking or when holding a posture such as with the arms outstretched in front of the body. The tremor can also affect the head, voice, legs, and trunk. Some people even feel an internal shake.

[5] www.hopkinsmedicine.org/

[6] Medline Plus.gov

[7] WebMD.com

[8] Perlmutter, David. Grain Brain. Little, Brown and Company (2013) Kindle Edition location 3041.

Chapter Ten

[1] Facebook group Essential Tremors - Self Help and Support - Greg's Story.

[2] The Great Courses.com Stress and Your Body.

[3] Taylor, Tina. Stress Effects: A fascinating look at the effects of stress on breathing patterns, gut microbiome, adrenals and addiction. Kindle Edition. Loc 342, 1222.

[4] Perlmutter, David. Grain Brain. Little, Brown and Company (2013) Kindle Edition Ch. 3.

[5] Taylor, Tina. Stress Effects. Kindle Edition. Loc 1222.

[6] Taylor, Tina. Stress Effects: Kindle Edition. Loc 340.

[7] Taylor, Tina. Stress Effects: Kindle Edition. Loc 369.

[8] Taylor, Tina. Stress Effects: Kindle Edition. Loc 391-400.

[9] mwkworks.com/desiderata.html

[10] Vitry, Loris. Breathe like a master! The anti-stress breathing technique for your healing. Kindle Edition. Loc 310-327.

[11] English, Paul. Sleep: 7 Ways to The Revolutionary Lifestyle. Kindle Edition. Loc 280.

[12] Presley, Elvis. quotefancy.com/quote/8181/Elvis-Presley-When-things-go-wrong-don-t-go-with-them.

[13] Wittmann, William. Playful Stress Reducing Shortcuts: Fast Drug-Free Ways to Tickle Your Nervous System to Improve Your Happiness, Peace, and Vitality. Kindle Edition. Loc 481, 491, 509.

Chapter Eleven

[1] Heather, Rose. 7 Top Anxiety Management Techniques: How You Can Stop Anxiety And Release Stress Today. Speedy Publishing LLC. Kindle Edition. Loc 37.

[2] Heather, Rose. 7 Top Anxiety Management Techniques: Kindle Edition.

Loc 324, 409, 475.

[3]Hooper, Jennifer. How to Deal With Anxiety: An interim Guide. Self Published. Kindle Edition. Loc 76-101.

[4]Pollan, Michael. How to Change Your Mind. Penguin Publishing Group. Kindle Edition. P. 41-74.

Chapter Twelve

[1]http://www.mayoclinic.org/diseases-conditions/tinnitus/symptoms-causes/syc-20350156

[2]Peters, Rose. TINNITUS the Thief of Silence: The lonely, hidden stress of never ending sound (The Self-Help Series Book 1). Kindle Edition. Loc 24, 160.

[3]www.cdc.gov/nceh/hearing_loss/public_health_scientific_info.html

[4]www.cdc.gov/nceh/hearing_loss/public_health_scientific_info.html

[5]www.enthealth.org/conditions/tinnitus/

[6]www.ncbi.nlm.nih.gov/pmc/articles/PMC1160568

[7]www.audicus.com/hearing-loss-and-musical-hallucinations/

[8]scholarworks.uark.edu/cgi/viewcontent.cgi?article=1059&context=rhrcuht

[9]Peters, Rose. TINNITUS the Thief of Silence: Kindle Edition. Loc 149.

Chapter Thirteen

[1]Stephens, Sasha. The Effortless Sleep Method. Kindle Edition. Loc 937

[2]Parsley, Kirk. Sleep to Win. Kindle Edition. Loc 370

[3]en.wikipedia.org/wiki/Ritual

[4]Baird, Chris. Sleep: Easy Sleep Solutions. Kindle Edition. Loc 686

[5] Bryan, Luis. Great Night's Sleep. Kindle Edition. Loc 229

[6]Nejad, Lillian. LIFEBLOCKERS The Sleep Edition. Kindle Edition. Loc 198

Chapter Fourteen

[1]Perlmutter, David. Grain Brain Little, Brown and Company. Kindle Edition. Loc 3009.

[2]http://www.nimh.nih.gov/health/topics/depression/index.shtml

[3]Firth. Frontiers of Psychiatry 15 May 2019. What Is the Role of Dietary Inflammation in Severe Mental Illness? A Review of Observational and Experimental Findings. P. 2 & 4.

[4]Firth. Frontiers of Psychiatry 15 May 2019. What Is the Role of Dietary Inflammation in Severe Mental Illness? A Review of Observational and Experimental Findings. P. 1.

[5]Perlmutter, David. Grain Brain Little, Brown and Company. Kindle Edition. Loc 3041.

[6]Firth, Joseph. Frontiers of Psychiatry 15 May 2019. What Is the Role of Dietary Inflammation in Severe Mental Illness? A Review of Observational and Experimental Findings. P. 6.

[7]http://www.mayoclinic.org/healthy-lifestyle/nutrition-and-healthy-eating/in-depth/mediterranean-diet/art-20047801

[8]Perlmutter, David. Grain Brain Little, Brown and Company. Kindle Edition.

[9]Firth, Joseph. Frontiers of Psychiatry 15 May 2019. What Is the Role of Dietary Inflammation in Severe Mental Illness? A Review of Observational and Experimental Findings. P. 6.

[10]Perlmutter, David. Grain Brain Little, Brown and Company. Kindle Edition. Loc 254.

[11]Firth, Joseph. Frontiers of Psychiatry 15 May 2019. What Is the Role of Dietary Inflammation in Severe Mental Illness? A Review of Observational and Experimental Findings. P. 7.

[12]Craft, Lynette. The Benefits of Exercise for the Clinically Depressed 2004 Prim Care Companion J Clin Psychiatry. P. 1

[13]Theron, Marcus. Anxiety: Rewire Your Brain Using Neuroscience to Free Yourself from Anxiety (Contains 2 Manuscripts: Rewire Your Brain & Use Neuroscience to Overcome Anxiety). Kindle Edition. Loc 547.

[14]www.health.harvard.edu/mind-and-mood/exercise-is-an-all-natural-treatment-to-fight-depression

Chapter Fifteen

[1]www.facebook.com/groups/188772458215430/

[2]www.ncbi.nlm.nih.gov/pubmed/27638063

[3]www.mayoclinic.org/drugs-supplements/propranolol-oral-route/side-effects/drg-20071164

[4]www.drugs.com/sfx/primidone-side-effects.html

[5]www.hopkinsmedicine.org/health/treatment-tests-and-therapies/home-epley-maneuver

Chapter Sixteen

[1]Yairi, Ehud. Epidemiology of Stuttering: 21st Century advances. P. 3.

[2]Yairi, Ehud. Epidemiology of Stuttering: 21st Century advances. P. 2.

[3]Yairi, Ehud. Epidemiology of Stuttering: 21st Century advances. P. 7.

[4]www.facebook.com/groups/188772458215430/

[5]Perez, Hector, Stuttering: Clinical and Research Update. P. 3

[6]www.reddit.com/r/Stutter/comments/3m4c59/marijuana_to_help_stuttering/

[7]https://www.scientificamerican.com/article/what-causes-stuttering-an/

Printed in Great Britain
by Amazon

19300494R00099